Routledge Revivals

International Studies
Volume 1

First published in 1931, this book is the first of three volumes that describe the circumstances of medical work in several European countries at that time. Together, the three books look at public administration, local and national, in relation to the prevention of disease. This first volume focuses on the Dutch, Scandinavian and German speaking countries, as well as Switzerland. It shows that many of these countries have gone beyond most others in the socialization of medicine, in several ways.

T0188339

International Studies
Volume 1
Prevention and Treatment of Disease

Sir Arthur Newsholme

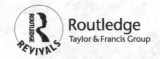

Routledge
Taylor & Francis Group

First published in 1931
by George Allen & Unwin

This edition first published in 2015 by Routledge
2 Park Square, Milton Park, Abingdon, Oxon, OX14 4RN
and by Routledge
711 Third Avenue, New York, NY 10017

Routledge is an imprint of the Taylor & Francis Group, an informa business

© 1931 Arthur Newsholme

Publisher's Note
The publisher has gone to great lengths to ensure the quality of this reprint but
points out that some imperfections in the original copies may be apparent.

Disclaimer
The publisher has made every effort to trace copyright holders and welcomes
correspondence from those they have been unable to contact.

A Library of Congress record exists under LC control number: 32001245

ISBN 13: 978-1-138-91256-4 (hbk)
ISBN 13: 978-1-315-69184-8 (ebk)
ISBN 13: 978-1-138-91263-2 (pbk)

INTERNATIONAL STUDIES

ON THE RELATION BETWEEN THE

PRIVATE & OFFICIAL PRACTICE *of* MEDICINE

WITH SPECIAL REFERENCE TO

THE PREVENTION OF DISEASE

conducted for

THE MILBANK MEMORIAL FUND

by

Sir ARTHUR NEWSHOLME
K.C.B., M.D., F.R.C.P.

Volume One

THE NETHERLANDS, SCANDINAVIA
GERMANY, AUSTRIA
SWITZERLAND

LONDON: GEORGE ALLEN & UNWIN LTD
BALTIMORE: THE WILLIAMS & WILKINS COMPANY

FIRST PUBLISHED IN 1931

FOREWORD

ON BEHALF OF THE MILBANK MEMORIAL FUND

ONE of the major problems in present-day public health administration is that of ascertaining the proper sphere of the private physician in the field of public health. Upon a number of occasions during the past few years this matter has been earnestly discussed by private physicians and public health administrators in joint assemblies arranged for the purpose, and some progress has been made in indicating what should be the relationship between private medicine and public health to ensure co-operative service in conserving the health of the public.

During the past seven years the Directors of the Milbank Memorial Fund have had occasion to consider this problem very seriously, in connection with the opposition of some members of the medical profession to certain phases of the public health work, which the Milbank Memorial Fund helped to inaugurate in one locality as a part of its participation in the New York State Health Demonstrations. This opposition led the Fund to re-examine the initial tenets upon which its participation in the health demonstrations was based, in order to make sure that its philanthropic service in the field of public health was not such as would in any way embarrass or impede fulfilment of the legitimate professional aspirations of the private medical practitioner. Finding in the history of public health development in the United States few precedents to guide them, the Directors decided to arrange for an international investigation to be made objectively and without bias, the purpose of the study being to throw light on the relationship in different countries between the fields of activity of private practising physicians and of physicians and laymen engaged in public health work. It was felt that studies of what was being done elsewhere in public health might be valuable in indicating not only solutions of problems, particularly affecting the relation between private physicians and physicians engaged in public health work, but specifically in showing how the co-operative services of private physicians may be utilised to the highest advantage by public authorities.

Such problems have arisen whenever preventive medicine has become in part clinical in character. In various countries medical treatment of the poorer members of the community is provided apart from private medical practice :

1. By the Poor Law authorities, for the destitute;
2. By voluntary organisations, in hospitals, dispensaries, and similar institutions, for those who are destitute in the sense of not being able to pay for specially skilled help;
3. Under public insurance schemes, which may be limited to medical aid or may also give financial assistance, and in which the State and the employer are, or may be, partially responsible, as well as the beneficiary;
4. By public health authorities, given at the expense of the taxpayer, as, for instance, in fever and smallpox hospitals and in sanatoria for tuberculosis, in venereal disease clinics, and to a smaller extent in maternity and infant consultation centres; and
5. By school or public health authorities in school clinics, at which eye defects, skin complaints, adenoids and tonsils, dental caries and other defects, are treated either gratuitously or at a small cost proportionate to the resources of the patient.

In different countries the activities under these and allied headings vary enormously. The public increasingly realises that each member of the community must have prompt and adequate medical care. By this means protraction of illness can be avoided, which in itself is a great public health gain; subsequent crops of such diseases as tuberculosis and the venereal diseases can be prevented; and the general standard of health and efficiency of the community can be raised.

As public health becomes more advanced and personal hygiene forms an increasing part of it, the stimulus to provide medical services either through voluntary or official organisations increases, and the delicacy of the relation

between private medical practitioners and voluntary and
official organisations becomes accentuated.

Hitherto, most countries have evolved measures for
reaching their hygienic objective only as each pressing
need has emerged. There has been irregular and unbalanced
progress, or stagnation has continued when opposition has
been severe. The different countries have not learned
adequately from each other; and at the present time, except
as regards insurance schemes in England and Germany,
but little international information of an accurate and
authentic character is available for the medical profession
and for social workers.

For the reasons incompletely set forth above, the Directors
of the Milbank Memorial Fund, in the summer of 1928,
secured the services of Sir Arthur Newsholme, M.D.,
K.C.B., former chief medical officer of the Local Government Board of England and Wales, and lecturer on public
health administration, School of Hygiene and Public
Health, the Johns Hopkins University, to make on their
behalf: (1) an objective study of what is being done for
the treatment as well as in the prevention of disease in the
chief European countries, including Great Britain and
Ireland; and (2) an impartial study of the philosophy of
the subject, with the hope that therefrom will emerge
further possibilities of action for the public good, which
are not inimical to the real interests of the medical
profession. The Directors of the Milbank Memorial Fund
are confident that the two interests are essentially identical; but they believe it important to base any con-
clusions and recommendations that may be reached on the
foundation of a wide and international investigation, which
has been objective in character. In securing the services of
Sir Arthur Newsholme to make the inquiries included in
this series, the Milbank Directors had confidence that his
long experience with the problems discussed in the studies
and his familiarity with conditions both in England and in
America qualified him to present an accurate account in
perspective of the pitfalls and triumphs of preventive

medicine and public health administration in the different countries concerned. It is understood, of course, that the Directors of the Milbank Memorial Fund in submitting herewith the findings of Sir Arthur Newsholme's international investigation do not commit the Fund to endorse his views in any respect or to approve the methods of public health work described. It is to be remembered that the essence of the investigation is to throw light on the relationship in different countries between practising physicians on the one hand, and physicians and authorities in public health work on the other hand; and this consideration explains the choice of subjects discussed in each chapter, which are selected as best illustrating this main problem.

JOHN A. KINGSBURY
Secretary

PREFACE TO VOLUME ONE

THIS volume, as already indicated in the introduction contributed by Mr. Kingsbury, on behalf of the Milbank Memorial Fund, is one of three similar volumes describing the circumstances of medical work in a number of European countries as related to public administration, local and national, when this concerns itself with direct measures for the prevention or treatment of disease.

The investigation, the results of which for a group of countries are here summarised, was undertaken to obtain a record of observed facts; and although here and there reflections on these facts have been made, the present and its companion volumes, except an independent volume dealing with general problems, maintain this limitation.

Evidently a survey of every branch of curative and preventive medicine is beyond the power of any single investigator, unless years were devoted to it, which would make the observations out of date before they were published. It has been necessary, therefore, to proceed by sampling these medical activities, selecting those which are typical or exceptional, and which are specially instructive to the workers engaged in medical administration or in private medical practice, who desire to have the light of experience in other fields thrown on their own problems.

Although the survey, as I have made it, is only partial, it may be claimed that much is gained from the fact that it has been made by one person only, and that the facts and observations embodied in it are thus fairly comparable. It may be added that the writer's familiarity for several decades with the task of selecting and assessing the salient features in actual public health problems has made his present task less laborious than it would otherwise have been, and has enabled him to select subjects concerning which an interchange of experience is most important.

My earliest inquiries in this investigation soon revealed the fact that in nearly every country visited by me almost identical difficulties were being experienced, some at their initial stages, in others partially solved; and ere long it became evident that these difficulties centred around certain specific medical problems. These are methods of medical attendance on the poor, the provision of hospital treatment and consultative facilities for the sick, the medical phase of sickness insurance, and the special problems of maternity and child welfare work, of school medical work, and of work for the treatment and prevention of tuberculosis and venereal diseases. In nearly every country it is concerning these problems that the "snags" of private medical practice in relation to the organised community recur and recur; and, although other aspects of medical work are not ignored, when points of interest emerge, it is to the study of the practice in regard to the above-mentioned problems that the following pages are chiefly devoted.

In order to understand the medical problems in each country studied, it has been found necessary to outline the governmental methods of the country concerned. Without this the administrative details of medical work would lose much of their significance.

In the present volume a specially interesting group of countries—the Dutch, the Scandinavian, and the German-speaking countries, and Switzerland—are placed under review. As will be seen by the prefatory summary to each chapter, some of these countries have gone beyond most other countries in the socialisation of medicine in one or another respect; and a study of the details of this movement has important bearings on the general problems behind the present investigation.

These general problems will be discussed in a separate volume, in which the experience in the different countries studied will be compared, and an attempt will be made to derive some general principles of action from the survey embodied in the preceding volumes.

It should be added that the contents of each chapter in this volume have been carefully revised in each instance by an important medical official of the country concerned. Although in each chapter I have expressed my indebtedness to the chief officials concerned, I must here more generally voice my gratitude for unsparing help and corrections, which enable me with confidence to pass the following pages for the press. If any mistakes have been made, I am personally responsible.

ARTHUR NEWSHOLME

January 1931

TABLE OF CONTENTS

CHAPTER V

GERMANY

CHAPTER VI

AUSTRIA

CHAPTER VII

INTERNATIONAL STUDIES

CHAPTER I

THE NETHERLANDS[1]

PRELIMINARY SUMMARY

This prosperous country is characterised by the predominantly voluntary and contributory character of its medical provision for a larger part of its population. Nearly every worker belongs to a sick fund. Of these funds there are many varieties; but they agree in one particular. Medical benefit is the only or the chief benefit, usually the only benefit. Commonly independent insurance for hospital treatment is also taken out. In some sick funds it is included with the medical benefit. The conditions of payment of doctors vary.

Midwifery is carried on chiefly by midwives, who in most districts are private practitioners. The training of midwives is restricted to the number needed in the country. Their training occupies three years.

Puerperal mortality in The Netherlands is very low. For discussion as to the degree of trustworthiness of puerperal statistics, see p. 41.

NATIONAL CONDITIONS

The Netherlands[2] is low-lying and flat, and intersected with canals. Much of it is below the sea-level. It is a country of agriculture and horticulture; but also has extensive interests in commerce and navigation, partly in connection with its extensive and well-managed colonies.

[1] Date of investigation, February 1929.
[2] Although frequently spoken of as "Holland" the official name for the whole country is The Netherlands, North and South Holland being two provinces of The Netherlands,

GOVERNMENT

Notwithstanding the old-world possession by its provinces and municipalities of extensive autonomous powers, events since the French Revolution have led to much greater centralisation and to curtailment of local powers. The Crown's consent is required for many local functions, and both the royal commissioner, who presides over each provincial council, and the burgomaster, who presides over each communal council, are appointed by the Sovereign.

The central Parliament of The Netherlands has an Upper and a Second Chamber. The former consists of fifty members, not elected by the people, but indirectly by the Provincial States for six years, half of them retiring every three years by rotation.

The Second Chamber is composed of one hundred Deputies, elected directly by universal bisexual suffrage on a system of proportional representation for four years. Locally The Netherlands is divided into eleven provinces and 1,081 communes. Each province has its representative body—Provincialen Staten (Provincial States)—elected for four years. All its members (which vary from thirty-five to eighty-two) retire together. The States can make ordinances affecting the welfare of the province and can raise local taxes, subject to the endorsement of the Crown. A royal commissioner (Commissaris), appointed by the Crown, presides over the provincial council, and exercises general authority in the province, in the half-yearly intervals between meetings of the State. He is guided in the conduct of detailed work by a provincial executive (Gedeputeerde Staten) of four to six members appointed by the Provincialen Staten.

Each of the 1,081 communes (Gemeente), whether urban or rural, large or small (several have a population under 500), is under a communal council (Raad), elected by proportional representation for four years, the number of representatives varying from seven to forty-five. This Raad can make and enforce by-laws affecting the common welfare, subject to Crown veto, and can raise local taxes. A central financial allowance comes from State taxation according to population. The local budget requires the approval of the provincial executive.

The local burgomaster is appointed by the Crown. He holds office for six years, and is usually reappointed. He has some independent executive power, especially as head of the police. He receives a salary and is pensionable. The executive work of the council is undertaken by the Collegiumvan Burgemeester en Wethonders (College of Burgomaster and Aldermen), and commonly certain branches of administration are assigned to individual aldermen.

There is somewhat active supervision of local administration by the Central Government.

The Minister of Labour, Commerce, and Industry is also Minister of Health. The present tenant of this office is Minister Slotemaker de Bruine, to whom, and his staff, I am indebted for much help in securing local information.

The Central Council of Public Health was established in 1902, to advise the Government not only on technical points, but also on the general direction of official control. Its president is Dr. Josephus Jitta, the general director of the public health service. There are five chief official inspectors who are *de jure* members of the Central Council.

These inspectors are allotted definite functions of supervision over local sanitary and medical work. One is concerned with medical practice, including the medical care of the poor and the control of infectious diseases. A second is concerned with pharmacy, foods, and drugs, and with water supplies; a third with housing; a fourth with the enforcement of the regulations for controlling the inspection of foods; and the fifth with the control of tuberculosis and venereal diseases. These inspectors have sectional assistant inspectors for divisions of the country. In addition, there are special inspectors of law enforcement as to alcoholic drinks and the supervision of subsidised societies and institutions.

The Central Council consists altogether of seventy mem-

bers, some nominated, others selected as specialists. The
unofficial members are unpaid, and the system is com-
mended as being economical! It must, I think, unless skilfully
managed, act as a clog on prompt and necessary official
activities.

There are somewhat similar local health commissions for
all populations over 18,000. These are nominated by the
Governor of the province on the recommendation of the
College of Aldermen.

The popularly elected municipal council is expected to
submit to the local health commission all resolutions passed
by them concerning health; but this, I am told, is not
always done. Any resolutions passed by the health commission may or may not be adopted by the municipal council.

The Central Government controls the central public
health laboratory and the serological institute through the
central health council and its chairman. At the laboratory
at Utrecht all the laboratory work required by the central
health council, by the inspectors of the Government and
the local health commissions is carried out. As a rule, no
charge is made for examinations of pathological specimens
submitted for diagnosis; but the cost may be, and is,
recovered from the well-to-do.

Special work for *child welfare* and for *medical inspection
of school children* has been relatively little developed in
The Netherlands, in marked contrast to the important
midwifery organisation.

Compulsory school attendance begins at six and ends
at twelve. Many children also attend nursery schools. At
Leyden there are four school doctors, engaged also in
private practice, whose visits are rather general inspections
than examination of individual children. In this university
town many of the defects of children are treated at the
public hospital of the medical school.

In Amsterdam there is a fuller school medical service,
each child being examined soon after admission to school.
There are two later less complete examinations of children.
Private doctors are informed of defects ascertained. Except

to a limited extent, as in the case of correction of defects of the teeth, treatment by the public service is in an early stage of development.

MEDICAL CARE OF THE POOR

Medical assistance in The Netherlands is not regarded as a state or provincial function. Like help for the poor in other respects, it is limited to instances in which voluntary organisations do not suffice. Religious bodies are active, both in giving medical and general relief; but, especially in towns, action by the municipality has become increasingly necessary. Speaking generally, arrangements for medical relief, while varying greatly, are ill-developed.

There is approximately one doctor to 2,000 inhabitants in The Netherlands, or 3,827 for its population of seven and a half millions. Medical studies are pursued at three universities (Leyden, Utrecht, Groningen), and at one municipal medical school (Amsterdam). The student's course is continued over six to seven years.

In Amsterdam persons too poor to belong to societies of medical help are treated by four semi-official doctors belonging to four divisions of the city. With such exceptions, non-institutional medical treatment for the poor is undertaken in The Netherlands by what would be called "club doctors" in Britain.

THE SICK FUNDS (CAISSES)

Nearly the entire wage-earning population of The Netherlands belongs to societies of medical help; but each person is left with the obligation of making his own provision for medical aid, including hospital treatment. The chief exception to this statement consists in the somewhat exiguous medical care of the destitute, for which the municipalities are responsible.

The responsibility has been met, as indicated above, by voluntary insurance, for which very numerous private enterprises and societies provide. Such funds existed long ago: in Delft, for instance, they date from 1603, 1622, and 1656, in connection with its guilds; their character is indicated by their names, such as "The Linen Weavers' Fund", St. Michael's or "The Broom-makers' Fund", and St. Crispin's or "The Shoemakers' Fund".

Gradually the need for similar arrangements and their potential advantages were realised; and action was taken, particularly in two directions: by employers who were anxious that their workers should have medical aid, including medicines; and by doctors and druggists, these acting individually or in co-operation with others, who thus became purveyors of medical treatment. Gradually the possibilities of financial gain by organising medical clubs were realised. Now many varieties of societies for medical help exist.

1. General societies with local branches.
2. Sick fund companies, which are on a commercial basis.
3. Funds managed by the employers of workmen or clerks; e.g. for factories, mines, railways, trams, managed by, or on behalf of, the directors.
4. Benevolent funds, catering for those near the point of destitution.
5. Mutual benefit funds, founded and carried on by the insured themselves.
6. Funds organised by doctors or by associations of doctors.
7. Other types.

The first of these are under the Society for Promoting Medicine. They work on centralised lines of organisation, with local branches all over the country; the local committee consists of equal numbers of doctors, druggists, and the insured.

The sick fund companies are organised similarly; they employ inspectors and agents, to canvass for subscribers.

In the industrial funds organised by employers, membership is compulsory for wage-earners, for other employees it is optional.

Benevolent funds are founded mostly by religious bodies for the benefit of their poorer members.

The mutual funds, founded and organised by workers, are often organised by political or religious parties or by large syndicates. They are run by committees of their members, trustees being appointed.

In larger towns socialist labourers have formed large societies. Doctors do not like these organisations because, in any dispute, the doctor's statement is liable to be disregarded.

Among other funds is one founded by the Society for Promotion of the General Good, the object of which is to defray the cost of medical attendance and death at a minimum rate, weekly subscriptions being paid on this basis.

The funds founded by doctors and druggists have a similar aim. Not the least interesting are those often arranged in smaller villages and the smaller towns. The doctor in a small village finds it advantageous to form his own society. The inhabitants pay their weekly sums to him. He thus ensures payment and they ensure treatment. In smaller towns often doctor, druggist, and secretary form a society.

The upper limit of wages of those who can become members of any of the above societies varies in different parts of the country. It has been raised considerably since the Great (World) War. It varies for families from 1,200, 1,600, and 1,800 to 2,000 guilders (guilder = 1s. 8d., or about 40 cents in the United States). In some societies more highly paid persons are admitted. The upper limit may also be raised for large families.

For single persons the upper limit is commonly set somewhat lower than the above. In some societies there is no maximum, or it may be settled for each individual case.

Membership in the religious, political, and industrial societies is limited by beliefs or by occupational restrictions. Industrial societies usually do not insure the worker's family; the only exception to this rule is the Railroads' Sick Fund.

On the other hand, the general societies commonly stipulate that a man cannot be a member unless his wife joins with him; as a rule, also children must be included.

In sick fund companies a member must be in good health when he joins.

The membership of these various societies varies from a few score up to 44,000 subscribing members, with a total membership of 80,000, which is the membership of the Co-operative Fund "De Volharding" (Perseverance) at The Hague.

The subscription varies greatly, in accordance with the extent of possible benefits. For families it is commonly 0·30 guilder (sixpence or 12 American cents), 0·40 guilder or 0·50 guilder a week, sometimes a little more. As a rule, no charge is made for children under sixteen years old; an additional premium is required for older children. This is generally half the above amounts, which is also the charge for single persons.

In some societies 5 or 8 cents (100 cents = a guilder) are charged for each child up to the age of sixteen.

Subscriptions are collected by the officials of each fund; and they may be payable at fixed hours and dates at the club rooms of the society. In industrial societies the subscription is deducted from wages.

The officials who collect subscriptions are paid on the basis of 5 to 10 per cent. of the amounts collected by them, or a fixed sum per member, or a weekly salary, the last-named method being adopted by the more important funds.

Members of organising committees are usually only paid out-of-pocket expenses, except the directors of sick fund companies.

After necessary expenses have been paid, the balance is disposed of in accordance with the special scheme of each fund. It may be divided between the doctors and druggists concerned; or these may be paid a fixed tariff per family or per member per annum.

The railroad funds pay a definite annual salary. Often druggists are paid at a fixed sum per prescription.

The chief benefit in each fund is medical aid, including surgical dressings. In special instances free obstetrical aid is supplied. Some of the more important societies provide free specialist aid, and supply spectacles, trusses, elastic stockings, flatfoot soles, etc. Others include dental aid and hospital nursing in their benefits.

There does not appear to be a free choice of doctors, or of midwives or druggists, except possibly within the limit of those employed by the particular fund. The rules vary, but the doctors of the society must be employed. The relation between the doctors and other officers and the fund is the subject of an agreement and rules. In large societies the maximum number of patients per doctor is fixed at 2,500 adults, and at 6,000 for the druggist.

In large towns it is usual for sick funds to form a league, in order to arrive at uniform methods so as to reduce expenditure on administration.

The Government at the present time is engaged in preparing legislation for regulating sick funds, and stating the conditions which they should fulfil.

Accident Insurance is entirely at the expense of the employer, who is required to pay 70 Dutch cents weekly for each person employed by him. This insures also for an old-age pension. A new law has been suggested which would provide that the employer should not be required to pay for insurance against accident, unless the employee belongs to a sickness insurance society.

HOSPITAL ORGANISATION

Hospital treatment is also the subject of insurance either in connection with sick funds or independently. The law requires municipalities to provide hospital treatment for the very poor; but there is increasing demand for hospital treatment for the poorer section of the self-supporting population, for whom it is ordinarily too costly, when needed without previous insurance. No law regulates the provision of hospital treatment, though efforts have been made in this direction; and now in increasing numbers the people are organising co-operative hospital insurance. The premium required is relatively small, from 7 to 10 cents a week for adults, less for children. This provides for maintenance and hospital treatment during thirty to sixty days, and partially, but only partially, for surgical aid, X-ray examinations, and transport. In Leyden one-half of the population contributes to this system of self-help, which is rapidly spreading over the country. In the larger towns this system has not existed until very recently.

Hospitals have first-, second-, and third-class patients, the first being treated in single-bedded rooms, the second in bedrooms with two beds, and the third in general wards. The third class is free for members of many sick funds, as well as to those subscribing to the special hospital insurance. There may be some payment, but reduced, for special treatment requiring spectacles, dentures, etc.

The Netherlands has hospital accommodation amounting to about three beds per 1,000 population. Four of its hospitals, with from 1,100 to 1,260 beds, are used by the State in medical teaching. In 1922 there were admitted into hospitals as patients a little over 2 per cent. of the population. The proportion of beds in different provinces varies from 0·7 to 4·8 per 1,000 of population.

Municipalities, to fulfil their legal obligation to provide hospital treatment for the poor, often contract with Presbyterian or Roman Catholic organisations for beds in the hospitals which these maintain.

Both hospital and domiciliary treatment of disease requires the assistance of nurses and of transport (ambulance) arrangements, and in securing these the "Crosses" of Netherland do valuable work. Their activities are multiform and on a very large scale. The Green Cross (Croix Verte) is the largest of them, having eleven provincial associations, 868 sections, and nearly half a million members. Its subscriptions in a year are not less than one and one-half million of Netherland florins or guilders. Its earliest activities were in securing home nursing; latterly it has undertaken much teaching of hygiene. In the Amsterdam section of The Netherlands the Croix Blanche preceded it. Both organisations play a similar rôle, and now they are federated. Their main object is to make home treatment approximate as nearly as possible to the efficiency of hospital treatment.

The Croix Blanche et Jaune Associations are Roman Catholic. They have 140 branches.

In all the three "Crosses" a chief point is to provide what are known in England as district nurses. There are altogether 600 nursing centres, of which 450 are "run" by the Croix Verte. In addition to their general nursing work, local tuberculosis associations are conducted almost exclusively by the Green and White Cross Societies, as also are convalescent homes. There is an elaborate ambulance system for conveying patients to hospital. Patients, unless insured, except the very poor, are required to pay for the ambulance.

THE TREATMENT OF TUBERCULOSIS

The main tuberculosis work is done by the sick funds, the "Crosses", and the anti-tuberculosis associations. Private initiative predominates, and this may be said to be the general characteristic of Dutch medical arrangements, if the word "private" be held to include all arrangements apart from those of the municipal or central government. There is no obligatory notification of cases of tuberculosis. In 1925 the mortality from phthisis was 0·70, and from other tuberculoses 0·29, per 1,000 of population.

There are between 500 and 600 anti-tuberculosis associations, to which the State usually contributes 5 Dutch cents per head of population if the commune adds another 5 cents. The State subvention is made conditional on examination by the doctor of the tuberculosis dispensary of each candidate for admission to a sanatorium.

A special diploma is given to those nurses who have qualified as tuberculosis visitors. There are thirty sanatoria in The Netherlands, with 4,800 beds, or about one to 2,800 persons. The proportion in Denmark is stated to be one in 1,900 (quoted from Dr. R. N. M. Eijkel's article in *L'Organisation Sanitaire des Pays-Bas*, League of Nations' publication, 1924). Patients in sanatoria as a rule contribute to their maintenance in the institution. One is struck with the multiplicity of agencies engaged in The Netherlands in anti-tuberculosis work, and a larger element of official unification of effort appears to be desirable.

THE TREATMENT OF VENEREAL DISEASES

Here again there is some State subvention, but on a relatively small scale. There are free clinics for these diseases in Rotterdam and Amsterdam, and at the university medical centres of Leyden, Utrecht, and Groningen. At the Rotterdam clinic sailors of all countries are treated gratuitously. Amsterdam has three venereal disease dispensaries. At several dispensaries advice is given on the basis of a medical prenuptial examination.

Organised medical effort to treat and control venereal disease is less general for venereal disease than for tuberculosis.

GENERAL CONSIDERATIONS

The Netherlands is a country in which private mutual medical organisation for the treatment of disease has been developed to an exceptional extent. This has been done without the ordinary sickness insurance which, in other countries, provides partial monetary support, in addition to medical aid.

The system in The Netherlands provides elementary medical attendance for the mass of the population. It cannot be doubted that the service could be improved and extended, if the different societies were to combine, and if the Government were to decide to assist in a more complete national organisation.

Meanwhile one must express admiration of the vast extent of voluntary co-operation in organising medical attendance. This could, I think, be retained, and rendered more effective with a simplified national scheme.

The special feature of medical work in The Netherlands —the feature which especially deserves study and, in many particulars, imitation—consists in its midwifery arrangements, which are fully described in the following section.

THE MIDWIFERY SERVICE

The attendance on midwifery cases in The Netherlands is very largely in the hands of exceptionally well-trained midwives; and as this arrangement is associated with a recorded mortality from puerperal sepsis and from other complications of pregnancy and confinement which is exceptionally low, the circumstances in The Netherlands call for detailed consideration.

Some tabular information may conveniently be stated at this point.

In 1928 there were 3,827 doctors, 919 midwives, and 487 dentists practising in The Netherlands.

According to official returns, the proportion to population of doctors, midwives, and dentists in four great towns is as shown in the accompanying table:—

POPULATION PER PRACTISING DOCTOR, MIDWIFE, OR DENTIST IN FOUR CITIES OF THE NETHERLANDS AND AVERAGE IN THE NETHERLANDS AS A WHOLE

Locality	Population per Each		
	Doctor	Midwife	Dentist
Amsterdam ..	1,179	6,024	6,073
Rotterdam ..	2,042	6,354	11,913
The Hague ..	913	9,047	4,955
Utrecht	770	13,787	4,214
The Netherlands ..	1,777	7,878	11,643

The number of midwives is restricted to about 900, or one per 8,000 of population. In The Netherlands as a whole some 40 per cent. of confinements are attended by doctors and 60 per cent. by midwives. The proportion of cases attended by doctors varies in different communes from 17 to 65 per cent.

The training of midwives in The Netherlands is exceptionally thorough and prolonged, as is also that of doctors. In a contribution in *L'Organisation Sanitaire des Pays-Bas*, 1924, published by the League of Nations, Dr. C. Meuleman, Director of the School of Midwives at Beerlen, gives interesting particulars comparing this training with that of other countries; and to this paper, and still more to Dr. Horst, the health officer of Leyden, I am indebted for the information summarised in the following pages.

In some countries six months' training has been regarded as adequate; and this was formerly so in England, though the training must now continue for a year, a period which is halved for fully trained nurses. In France and Belgium two years' training is demanded (but see Vol. II); in The Netherlands the period is three years.

In all schools for midwives substantially the following course is followed:—

First, all the candidates must possess a good education and pass a severe preliminary examination. Then there follows a course of training during three years, for which there are three schools, one of these being conducted by Roman Catholics. The course of training is very practical, and is controlled by professors of obstetrics and gynæcology.

The preliminary examination comprises the writing of an essay, the solution of some arithmetical problems, and answers to questions in physical science. In the oral examination, questions in history, geography, and physics are asked. Much stress is laid on the intelligence and carriage of candidates.

On entering the school each candidate is given a uniform, resembling that of a nurse. During the first three months courses of anatomy and physiology are followed, and the subjects of the preliminary examination are continued. Courses on hygiene are given by a member of the medical staff, continuing through three years. After three months theoretical lessons in obstetrics are given. The student also begins to help, to some extent domestically, in the clinic of the school. In the second year the student is admitted to the lying-in ward, and is instructed by means of the obstetric dummy, also as to the pathology of pregnancy, parturition, and the lying-in period. She is also entrusted with the nursing of healthy infants born in the clinic. Later in this second year she is allowed to conduct deliveries under the direction of the doctor or the chief midwife. At the end of this year the student passes her first examination. This examination includes the examination of a pregnant woman and the diagnosis of fœtal position, followed by tests with an artificial pelvis and fœtus; also *vivâ voce* questions on general hygiene and on the management of the infant.

During the third year the student works more frequently in the lying-in ward, and assists in the examination of pregnant women, and in special consultations for mothers and infants. She also helps the younger students. At the end of nine months of this third year she passes her final examination as a midwife. The director and medical professors of the school are her examiners. She still remains for three months at the school, or takes the place, during this time, of older midwives who come back to the school for a gratuitous post-graduate course of reinstruction. In Amsterdam and Rotterdam third-year pupils are allowed to practise in the town under the direction of midwives. The two Governmental schools of midwifery are free for students. At the Catholic school fees are paid.

The number of candidates allowed to undergo training is limited by Government regulations, so that the supply of midwives cannot become excessive. This is in sharp contrast to the training of doctors, in which the ordinary law of supply and demand holds good. Often there are thirty-five candidates for ten places in a midwifery school. The maintenance of the pupil midwives, as well as their teaching, is paid for by the Government. It may be added here that nurses must obtain a Government diploma, and cannot otherwise take the name of nurse, or wear the official emblem of a nurse. There is no diploma for home (health) visitors, and many women practise as nurses without a diploma and without the legal title of nurse.

Midwives are urged by Government officials to make a maximum charge of 15 guilders per case, while doctors are recommended to charge at least 25 guilders; and it has even been proposed to exercise disciplinary pressure on doctors through their own association to prevent them from charging less than this. The fear, in official quarters, appears to be that midwives may decrease in numbers, and efforts are directed to their maintenance.

The proportion of confinements attended by midwives varies greatly in different communities. The proportion varies to some extent according to the proportion of young doctors, older doctors wishing to withdraw from the practice of midwifery. Through doctors and midwives, the midwifery service is very complete. In 1909, out of 1,000 total births in The Netherlands, only 19 had no skilled help in confinement. There appears to be no evidence of difference in the proportion of still-births in midwives' and doctors' cases.

Midwifery by midwives is limited—as in England—to natural parturition. Only if no doctor is available can the midwife attend to complications, and even then she must not employ instruments. Occasionally when a doctor and a midwife are in somewhat competitive practice in the same district, the subordination of the midwife to the doctor in complicated midwifery has caused difficulties.

The law requires each commune to have a midwife. The municipality pays for the poorest mothers. Usually the midwife is paid a retaining fee, such that she can out of private practice make it up to the 1,800 guilders a year required to live.

As already stated, the midwife may not use forceps; but abandonment of this restriction is being mooted. She may administer ergotin according to regulations.

The midwife when attending a poor woman can claim the help of the local doctor for the poor (Gemeente-arts). This doctor usually is a local general practitioner, receiving a small salary for his work from the municipality. Persons not belonging to the real poor must pay for the doctor themselves. Usually they are members of a *fonds* (i.e. fund), which gives co-operative insurance for medical aid. To maintain membership of the *fonds* a regular payment of from 20 to 26 cents weekly is required. Evidently this arrangement is not so satisfactory from the midwife's and the patient's points of view as the English official plan, in which medical help—with a free choice of doctor—is made available for all without distinction on the call of the midwife; though the doctor's fees can be partially, or perhaps altogether, recovered from the patient or her husband at a later date. In The Netherlands, when specialists are not available, people almost invariably choose the doctor who attends the family in ordinary illness.

In the university town of Leyden somewhat special conditions exist. The municipality retains three midwives for the poor at a salary of 300 guilders a year (a guilder is 1s. 8d.), but they have very little work. Advanced medical students attend nearly all the confinements among the poorer classes, "baker" (mostly trained nurses or women with a special training for this work only) assisting the student at the confinement or afterwards. All these work under the supervision of the professor. Every expectant mother making arrangements for her confinement must see the professor of gynæcology, who decides whether the patient shall be delivered in hospital or at home. The service given is gratuitous. In the other university towns of Amsterdam, Utrecht, and Groningen somewhat different conditions exist. In Amsterdam there are seventeen municipal midwives for the poor as well as independent midwives. The midwives give antenatal care to their own cases.

The urine is always examined, but blood pressure is not systematically taken. So far as the entire country is concerned, the question whether midwives shall be supplied with a blood-pressure outfit has arisen. Some of them already make this test.

The nurses who assist the medical students in Leyden belong to special organisations; and most of the mothers insure to receive their services.

The general impression I received from the many inquiries made by me was that the midwifery service in The Netherlands is exceptionally efficient and complete. The midwives are carefully selected and their preliminary educational standard is high. Their number is limited and selected from a large number of candidates. They receive training at the expense of the State, which stretches over three years, and includes practical work under a doctor or midwife.

The training of a medical student before he becomes qualified extends over seven years. Thus—and perhaps this is most important of all—the doctors who assist them in emergencies have had an exceptionally protracted students' career, allowing of adequate training in midwifery.

In midwifery their training is as follows: First, three years are occupied with preliminary studies of chemistry, physiology, anatomy, etc. Then they begin to attend the University Hospital. During this fourth year they have three hours weekly on the theory of obstetrics; one hour weekly on the obstetric dummy; and one hour weekly on gynæcology.

In the fifth year these same courses are continued to an equal extent. In the sixth year other branches of practical non-obstetrical work occupy the whole time.

In the seventh year the above courses are continued to the same extent; but an additional one and one-half hours are added for examination of pregnant women, exercises on the dummy, and studies on the pelvis, some microscopy (placenta, pathological products, etc.).

In the fifth year each student attends five confinements at the hospital, and before his final examination he must have attended fifteen confinements at home, of which at least two must be complicated cases (forceps or other). Also each student must assist in a group of six, as an onlooker, twice a week at various operations.

Since the above section was written I have received, through the courtesy of Dr. Horst, Medical Officer of Health of Leyden, the following contribution, which throws valuable additional light on midwifery arrangements in The Netherlands.

MIDWIVES IN THE NETHERLANDS

By S. Sievertsen Buvig

Mistress-Midwife at the State Training School for Midwives at Amsterdam

It affords me pleasure to accede to a request for some particulars regarding midwifery in Holland, and for the sake of completeness I shall commence with a short historical retrospect.

There was a time in this country when obstetrics was exclusively in the hands of midwives, whose knowledge in those early times was derived solely from practical experience.

Nevertheless it was at an early period in history that the vast importance to the health of the community of a well-instructed corps of midwives was recognised, and there are abundant signs to show that the authorities in the flourishing townships evinced the greatest interest as to their efficiency and system of training. It was made a rule that they should be under the superintendence of the local surgeons' guild, from which they received their certificate of efficiency. They were then entitled to set up as private midwives and to take pupils to whom, also under the superintendence of the guild, they imparted the requisite practical and theoretical knowledge and who, after completing a certain term of instruction, were called upon in their turn to give proofs of their skill before the guild.

This practical training held sway for a long time, but after a time the theoretical instruction was entirely reorganised, so that at the brightest period in our history, in the seventeenth century, when art and science flourished to an unprecedented degree, the instruction of the midwives was led into what, for those times, may be termed excellent lines. At that period there were men like Cornelius Solingen, who lived from 1641 to 1687, and Frederik Ruijsch, two of the greatest scholars of the seventeenth century in medical science, who thought it not beneath them to take an active interest in the instruction of midwives. This instruction was, by the nature of things, purely theoretical. The practical knowledge was acquired in practice. But, compared with the conditions prevailing in former times, it was undeniably an immense step forward. It was in those days that the first textbook for midwives was published in this country. It was a translation of the work of the famous German midwife, Justine Sigesmunden, and no one less than Professor Solingen himself supervised its adaptation.

THE TRAINING SCHOOL

For many years this state of matters continued, the instruction always being given by the most eminent men. In the course of time, however, the need was felt for putting the practical and the theoretical training into the same hands, and thus the idea originated of establishing special schools of midwifery. It was in 1861 that this stage was reached and the State Training School for Midwives founded at Amsterdam.

At first the school served merely to house the pupils. They obtained their theoretical lessons with the medical students at the clinical school, and the practical duties were performed at a lying-in ward which had meanwhile been instituted in connection with one of the hospitals and which was under the management of a mistress-midwife. This, then, was a further step forward—from this time the practical as well as the theoretical instruction was given by a professional. And so it has remained up to the present day, although in the course of years it was felt advisable to have all the instruction given in the same building. This was achieved in 1885, when thirteen pregnant women came to the school for their confinements. This number growing each year, the original building speedily became too small, and in 1900 the school was removed to its present quarters, which, however, since that date have been greatly enlarged, for the number of confinements has risen during the last few years to about one thousand.

When the School for Midwives was founded by the State, it was enacted that the training should continue two years. Five years ago the course was lengthened by one year, so that it now extends over a period of three years.

THE COURSE

Before being admitted to the training schools (there is one at Amsterdam and one at Rotterdam) candidates must pass an entrance examination before examiners appointed by the Government. The pupils must have had the usual school-board education. The examination, however, is competitive, so that as a rule the candidates are far above this standard. They are admitted in order of merit, and the total number of pupils divided over the three years' course is about forty to each school. All the pupils live in. The fees are two hundred Dutch florins per annum.

The instruction, which in the first year, is almost entirely theoretical, comprises anatomy, physiology, bacteriology, obstetrics, physics, and chemistry; while three hours per week during each of the three years are devoted to Swedish gymnastics.

The practical work is confined to domestic assistance in the lying-in wards, whereby the pupil becomes familiarised with the hospital sphere.

In the second year the practical work commences. Under the guidance of the mistress-midwife or one of her assistants the pupil has to conduct labours, to nurse patients, and to attend infants. Clinical lessons and practice with the "phantom" alternate with the purely theoretical lessons in obstetrics. The classes for physics and chemistry are continued, and it is made compulsory for the second-year pupils to reattend the first year's lessons by way of revision. At the end of this year an examination is held, the so-called first or theoretical part of the examination for midwife. If the candidate passes she is competent to conduct labours outside the clinic under the superintendence of a midwife.

In the third year the pupil works outside the school in order that she may become acquainted with the difficulties commonly met with in practice before her training is completed. She works thus in certain districts of the town under the superintendence of the municipal midwife in the respective districts. Further, the pupil also receives instruction in the third year in hygiene and in child welfare, besides acting as assistant at the consultation bureau for child welfare. At the end of nine months she has to undergo the final examination, but her connection with the school is not severed until the session is fully completed.

During the latter months the midwives who have finished their training are enabled to attend a course of recapitulatory classes, during which time their practical work is performed for them by the third-year pupils. This arrangement has the double advantage that the pupils gain practical experience, and the midwives are enabled to participate in these recapitulatory classes without pecuniary sacrifices.

It will be quite evident that when the pupil leaves the training-school she is excellently grounded both practically and theoretically.

THE PROFESSIONAL MIDWIFE

The time is long past when all labours were attended by midwives, though that is still the case in a few very country places. As a rule the midwife attends the poorer people and the doctor those in the more well-to-do classes.

Nevertheless, until a few years ago, about 75 per cent. of the births were attended by midwives. This was mainly due to the great disparity between the physician's and the midwife's charges. For about ten years, however, the possibility of obtaining a university education has become so much greater that our little country has now a superfluity of university graduates and likewise of doctors. This surplus has become so marked that we are justified in making use of the term "intellectual masses", as we formerly spoke of the "uneducated masses". The result of this is, however, that the supply of educated workers far exceeds the demand, and so, too, in the medical profession. Our country now has enough doctors for them to begin to compete with the midwives, so that, in recent years, fewer and fewer labours have been attended by the latter. The statistics show that during last year this number had fallen to about 60 per cent. of the whole.

Until these conditions are in some way regulated, the midwives will continue to have difficult times. Those who are best provided for at present are those in the service of a municipality, as is the case with some in Amsterdam. These receive a fixed salary, and have to attend labours as directed by the medical officer of health. But those whose work is so regulated are by far in the minority. The majority in the large towns are so-called "private midwives", who have set up in practice and who receive their fees from the patients.

In the smaller places and in the country the midwife generally receives an allowance from the municipality, and for each delivery she also gets a certain fee from the patient, according to her social position and the class of district in which she lives.

As regards her work, the midwife in Holland enjoys a liberty of action unknown elsewhere. She is only prohibited from using obstetric instruments, and bound, when necessary, to summon medical assistance, and she has the competency and the capacity to act herself in a case of emergency. This lays great responsibility on her, but renders the work peculiarly attractive to earnest women. It goes without saying that she has to watch over the childbed and to care for the infant. Further, in the training of the midwife great attention is paid to the observance of the gravida, and the midwife is thoroughly instructed as to what complications may arise. Especially is she trained how to recognise and prevent eclampsia. It is largely due to this fact that this complication is slowly disappearing in our country.

In conclusion I may say that the midwives have associated themselves into a society, the Union of Dutch Midwives, of which the majority of midwives are members. This association has its own organ, while there is also a special scientific Journal of Midwifery.

THE STATISTICS OF MATERNAL MORTALITY

Can the above favourable conditions in the midwifery service be related to an exceptionally low puerperal mortality? A partial answer to this question should be furnished by the national and district statistics of death from complications of pregnancy and parturition; and, were one quite certain that international comparisons are dependable, a definite answer might be given to the question.

Professor H. W. Methorst, the Director of the Centraal Bureau voor de Statistiek for The Netherlands, to whose help I am much indebted, supplied the data from which the following table has been made. The classification of puerperal mortality of the International List (numbers 143–150) is used in The Netherlands, the data being thus theoretically comparable with those of other countries. The deaths include sepsis (146), phlegmasia embolia (147), albuminuria (148), and other puerperal conditions (143, 144, 145, 149, 150).

These deaths in the accompanying table are given along with the number of live-births, and the rates compounded of the two. For Amsterdam, The Hague, and Leyden, the total puerperal deaths and death-rate alone are given, as the numbers concerned are small. I have given only the average

AVERAGE PUERPERAL MORTALITY IN THE NETHERLANDS, AND IN THREE CITIES OF THE NETHERLANDS, FOR THE FOUR YEARS 1924–27

Area	Population	Number of Puerperal Deaths	Number of Live-Births	Puerperal Death-Rate per 1,000 Live-Births
The Netherlands	7,625,938[1]	1923[2]	713,566	2·69
Amsterdam ..	734,884	190	55,311	3·61
The Hague ..	416,179	103	30,289	3·40
Leyden ..	69,851[1]	17	5,778	2·60

[1] Population in 1928.   [2] Of these, 600 were from puerperal septicæmia·

rate for the four years 1924–27, in order to reduce accidental variations. Certain points of doubt emerge. Registration of a birth in The Netherlands must take place within three days (not including holidays), and if a live-born child dies before the declaration of birth has occurred, such child is registered as *levenloos aangegeven* (declared lifeless). This would materially vitiate comparison between infant death-rates (per 1,000 live-births) in England and in The Netherlands, were comparisons to be made without having added to the number registered in The Netherlands the number of infants born alive but dying before registration; but so far as puerperal death-rates are concerned, the only influence of such a course would be to raise slightly the recorded puerperal mortality in that country. We may therefore ignore this point for puerperal mortality.[1] As already stated, there is international uniformity as to the morbid conditions named in death certificates which comprise puerperal mortality. There remains, however, the question as to whether the same practice is adopted in the statistical office in The Netherlands, as, for instance, in England and Scotland, in allocating or refraining from allocating to the puerperal heading deaths during pregnancy, or in connection with parturition. No uniform practice can be certainly said to be internationally followed. The English and Scottish rules for medical practitioners in signing certificates of death contain the following paragraph:—

Whenever parturition or miscarriage has been in any way a contributory cause of death, the fact should be mentioned on the certificates. Always qualify all diseases resulting from childbirth or miscarriage as puerperal, e.g. puerperal septicæmia, puerperal peritonitis, etc.

In England a statement of sepsis would lead to a death after confinement being returned under this heading, in preference to nearly all other causes of death except violence which might also be given on the same certificate, but no

[1] For statistics prior to 1924 the above statement is correct. From 1924 onward, infant birth-rates and death-rates in England, the United States, and The Netherlands are precisely comparable.

special preference in classifying is given to puerperal conditions other than sepsis.

In the United States (*Manual of Joint Causes of Death*, 1925) puerperal causes generally are preferred to influenza, when both are mentioned in the death certificate; whereas the English and Scottish rule would appear, in such a case, to prefer influenza even to puerperal sepsis in classifying. In 1918 the operation of the American rule was associated with a sudden rise of puerperal mortality. Had England followed this practice, the deaths officially ascribed to parturition would have been increased by ninety-six influenza deaths in 1925, while in 1918 the puerperal deaths would have been increased by 1,638! This illustration shows the occasional embarrassment which may arise through an exceptional preference in classification of the puerperal condition, when a pregnant or lying-in woman dies as the result of a presumably independent infectious disease. Of course, there is the likelihood that occasionally a true puerperal sepsis is returned as influenza when the English plan is adopted. Evidently the international position is somewhat chaotic; and it is doubtful if the chaos could be removed by the adoption of a rigid and detailed international system of rules, so much depending on the personal bias of the statistician responsible for relegating a dubious certificate embodying more than one item to its right compartment.

Meanwhile, unfortunately, with the same international rules for certification of causes of death, but with differences (*a*) in the extent to which recent parturition is mentioned in the death certification, and (*b*) in the practice in different countries as to the relative importance attached to various causes of death during the puerperium, it is possible to have considerable differences in puerperal death-rates which do not correspond with real differences in puerperal death-rates. This is illustrated by the English *Registrar-General's Review for 1925* (Text). This gives the certified cause of 2,900 deaths certified as being puerperal in origin, and, in addition, of 759 deaths of women in which the "causes of

death were stated to have been complicated by the existence
of the puerperal state". A few of the largest causes of death
thus coincident with the puerperal state are given in the
accompanying table:—

CAUSES OF DEATH IN WHICH THE PUERPERAL STATE
WAS GIVEN AS A COMPLICATING FACTOR FOR 759
WOMEN IN ENGLAND, 1925.

Primary Cause of Death	Number
Influenza	96
Respiratory tuberculosis ..	76
Pernicious anæmia	18
Cardiac valvular diseases ..	110
Other cardiac diseases.. ..	73
Pneumonia	127
Intestinal obstruction	24
Chronic nephritis	25
Miscellaneous diseases.. ..	210
Total	759

Evidently here is considerable opportunity for varying
practice. The association in such cases as the above may
be, and generally is, purely accidental, the normal physiological process of parturition not having contributed
to the lethal effect of an intercurrent disease. I do not
know of any country outside Britain which invites the
statement on a death certificate of associated parturition
or pregnancy.

I have set out these difficulties at this point because any
judgment as to international puerperal statistics must have
them constantly in mind. As the practice in England and
Scotland does not differ markedly, there can be little doubt
that the puerperal mortality rates for these two countries
may be compared. In the years 1921–27 it varied in England
and Wales for total puerperal mortality from 3·91 to 4·12,
and in Scotland from 6·2 to 6·4, per 1,000 live-births,

while that from puerperal sepsis in the same period varied in England from 1·30 to 1·60, and in Scotland from 1·64 to 2·03. Scotland has a rather higher birth-rate than England, and its higher puerperal mortality is therefore not explicable by a larger proportion of first-births, with the greater risk accompanying these.

Are The Netherland figures comparable with those for England and Scotland? Professor Methorst has favoured me with the following remarks, in answer to my question as to whether certifying doctors in The Netherlands are asked to state on the death certificate whenever the deceased had been delivered of a child within a month of death:—

In The Netherlands there are no prescriptions that certifying physicians should state the fact of parturition if this has occurred within a month before death; but as nearly every parturition is observed by a qualified physician or midwife, as every certificate of the cause of death must be signed by a qualified physician after personal inquest, there will be only few cases of death where connection with pregnancy, parturition, or childbed will escape attention or registration.

Moreover, every case of death is reported to the Central Bureau for Statistics, and the causes of death of each case pass —one by one—the control of the Medical Officer of the same office. In doubtful cases (for instance, peritonitis, sepsis, operation, hæmorrhage, thrombosis, and embolia, etc.) a letter is sent by same Medical Officer (qualified physician) to the declaring physician inquiring after possible connection with abortion, pregnancy, etc. These letters are hardly ever left unanswered.

In the following diagram I have compared the recorded experience of Scotland and of England and Wales, during the period 1921–27, with that of The Netherlands, and of three towns in it for the average of the years 1924–27. Even if it be assumed that in The Netherlands the fact of recent parturition remained unstated oftener than in Britain, it appears to me highly improbable that the real relative position of the three countries would be changed by corrections. In my view it is fairly certain that Scotland has a puerperal experience much less favourable than that of England; and that England's experience likewise is not nearly so satisfactory, in regard to puerperal mortality, as that of The Netherlands.

The diagram below shows that in the two largest towns of The Netherlands puerperal mortality is higher than in the country as a whole. This fits in with the similar excess

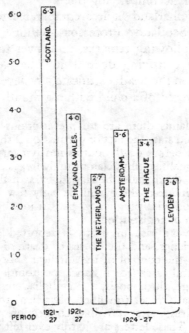

THE RATE OF TOTAL PUERPERAL MORTALITY IN THE NETHERLANDS AND ITS CHIEF TOWNS, COMPARED WITH THAT OF ENGLAND AND SCOTLAND.

in towns shown more or less in Scandinavian countries and in Germany. It may be due in part to the greater number of abortions in towns. The comparison in the diagram with England and with Scotland is instructive. I do not think that more than a relatively small part of the difference between Denmark and Great Britain can be ascribed to differences in the completeness of association of certified deaths with parturition.

CHAPTER II

DENMARK[1]

PRELIMINARY SUMMARY

In visiting Denmark one is impressed by the cleanliness and orderliness of its people, by the absence of indications of poverty, and by the fact that the evident prosperity of the country appears to be more evenly distributed than is found elsewhere.

Denmark presents many features of special medical interest. Its general hospitals, with special departments, attain a very high standard, and are probably more readily available and more completely utilised by the population than are their hospitals by any other people outside Scandinavia.

In bringing about this hospitalisation of treatment Denmark's systems of sickness and invalidity insurance have borne a great part. The first of these is unique, in that without introduction of compulsion the majority of the Danish population are insured. Denmark's sickness insurance deserves special attention also, in that it appears to work, as a rule, satisfactorily both to the insured and to the doctors, on whose fidelity and accuracy in certification as well as in medical treatment the success of sickness insurance must always depend.

Denmark, like the other Scandinavian countries, is important in that most of its obstetric work is done by midwives, without the evil results sometimes assumed to be inevitable when doctors do not have experience of normal midwifery in their ordinary practice.

Lastly, Denmark began 130 years earlier than Great Britain, and even earlier than other countries, a system of gratuitous treatment of venereal diseases throughout the country for all patients, irrespective of social or financial status. This, from the beginning, was associated with a corresponding obligation on the part of the patient to continue treatment until free from infection.

[1] Date of investigation, June 1930.

For the above, among other reasons, the institutions of Denmark and its people are supremely worthy of study by the physician, the hygienist, and the social worker. Its industries are equally interesting and important, as showing how a country with limited natural advantages—except its maritime position—has succeeded in becoming and remaining prosperous in spite of the national and economic obstacles incident to the martial and commercial struggles of the world outside Denmark.

GENERAL CONDITIONS

A short statement as to the topography and the industries of Denmark will help us to understand more clearly its successful co-operative work in the field of hygiene and medicine.

Denmark, including North Slesvig (added since the Great War), has an area of 42,900 square kilometres, and at the census of November 1925 had a population of 3,434,555, of whom 568 out of every 1,000 lived in rural districts. Its population about equals that of New Jersey or Missouri. Copenhagen, without its suburbs, had a population of 587,150.

The population is almost entirely Scandinavian, and this homogeneity of race—backed up by corresponding homogeneity of religion and education—partially explains the success of the various co-operative social activities named or described in the following pages. But this explanation is not adequate. Something must be ascribed also to its insular climate, which, like that of Great Britain, impels to enterprise at home and overseas. The innate characteristics coming down from the days of the Vikings of the eighth to the tenth century, which in earlier times showed themselves in raids and in piracy, must also be reckoned as actuating in large part the successful struggle in Denmark for economic and social well-being during the last sixty or seventy years.

At present Denmark's economic welfare is wrapped up chiefly with its exportation of bacon, butter, and eggs to

Great Britain. Denmark supplies one-third of the butter, one-fourth of the bacon, and over one-tenth of the eggs on the world export market.[1]

This wonderful growth of agricultural production has occurred since the eighties of the nineteenth century. In earlier years Denmark was an exporting wheat country; but as it could not compete with the cheap grain then arriving from overseas, it diverted its energies co-operatively in a new direction with marvellous success.

One cannot fail to see the ancient Northmen's spirit in this achievement; and a Briton may be excused for claiming for his countrymen—as also for all Anglo-Saxon people—a part in the same spirit of enterprise and of unwillingness to accept defeat. In the centuries preceding the Norman invasion of England, Danes and other Norsemen left a permanent impress on England and Scotland. They possessed without subsequent retreat much of the eastern part of Scotland and a large share of North-Eastern England. This is still seen in physical and mental characteristics common especially to the inhabitants of these parts of Great Britain and of the Scandinavian countries. It is not without interest that the Danish King of England, Canute or Knud, appears to have had before him the ideal of an Anglo-Scandinavian Empire, and he invaded Norway to this end.

Norway and Denmark have always been intimately inter-related; in the fourteenth century these two countries and Sweden were under one Government. It was not until 1814 that Norway was ceded to Sweden. More recently, Norway has "set up house" independently of Sweden; and the relation between the three Scandinavian countries now is very friendly.

The educational system of Denmark has been an important means towards economic success and social improvement. In addition to universal elementary education, which has been compulsory since 1814, there are also now technical

[1] See *Agriculture, the Co-operative Movement*, etc., in Denmark (League of Nations publication, 1929).

schools with 26,000 pupils, 21 training-colleges for teachers with 1,900 pupils, 93 commercial schools with 13,000 pupils. There are, furthermore, 21 agricultural schools with a yearly attendance of about 1,900 pupils, and 22 schools for housekeeping and domestic economics at which some 500 girls attend yearly. The People's High Schools (Grundtvig, Kold) are attended by pupils who have received the ordinary school education, the course in them lasting from three to nine months. They are largely subsidised by the Government. Attendance is voluntary, and these schools embody the principle of private management and Government supervision, with some control over expenditure, which, as will be seen shortly, runs through every field of Danish activity.

Along with the important work of the People's High Schools has gone the breaking up of the large estates of Denmark. Smallholdings, in which the labourer working for a wage has been largely replaced by the small proprietor who has a stake in the success of his farm, have taken the place of most of the larger farms. About 85 per cent. of Danish farms have an area of less than 30 hectares (about 74 acres); and 94 per cent. of the farms are freehold. Such smallholdings would probably spell permanent poverty had not the Danes showed a unique capacity to co-operate in their agricultural work. Agriculture is pre-eminently an individualistic occupation; it appears in some countries to be essentially inimical to co-operation; but Denmark has solved the problem by co-operative buying and selling. Local co-operative associations have been formed in every district for combined buying of seeds and implements, and for combined selling of all produce. In these associations the democratic principle has been rigidly followed, the small owner having an equal vote with the owner of a large estate. The local co-operative associations have united in national industrial enterprises, so that in most transactions the mutual benefits of buying and selling on a large scale are secured.

This co-operation in business has been rendered possible

by mutual respect and confidence, which have rendered it possible also, as seen hereafter, to co-operate on voluntary lines in medical provisions and in insurance against sickness without introducing the element of compulsion. In considering the genesis of these movements one must ascribe much importance to Denmark's educational system and to its co-operative associations in developing the sense of social integrity.

Dr. Boudreau[1] has pointed out also how the high standard of bacterial cleanliness and exactitude in methods of asepsis, and the coincident education of agriculturalists in the rôle of bacteria, have rendered easier the task of the hygienist than it would otherwise have been.

One may mention at this point the personal and domestic cleanliness which appears to be a general characteristic of the Danes. The significance of this in relation to safe child-bearing should not be lost sight of (p. 65).

I do not describe, hereafter, Denmark's important contribution to the prevention of tuberculosis from food products, as it is foreign to my main subject; but this has formed a valuable piece of international sanitary work.

Denmark's birth-rate in 1928 was 19·6 per 1,000 of population, while its crude death-rate was 11 per 1,000 of population; its tuberculosis death-rate was about 1 per 1,000; its infant mortality (1928) was 81 per 1,000 infants born alive. The last-named figure is somewhat excessive; and infantile diarrhœa still causes nearly 10 per cent. of all deaths of infants. Illegitimacy is somewhat high, about 10 per cent. of the births in Denmark occurring outside matrimony.[2] Divorce also is high. Infant mortality is lower both in Sweden and Norway than in Denmark.

GOVERNMENT

Legislative power lies jointly with the King and the Rigsdag (Diet). Executive power is vested in the King, who exercises it through his ministers.

[1] *Op. cit.*, p. 5.　　[2] *International Year Book of the League of Nations*, 1925.

The Rigsdag has two Houses—the Folketing (House of Representatives) and the Landsting or Senate.

The Folketing has 149 members, of whom 117 are elected by the method of proportional representation in 23 districts, while 31 additional members are divided among minority parties, and one member is elected for the Faroe Islands by simple majority.[1]

Of the members of the Landsting, 56 are elected by the voters for the Folketing who are over thirty-five years of age, 19 additional members being elected on a proportional basis by the previous Landsting. Members of the Landsting hold office for eight years, of the Folketing for four years, unless the King dissolves this assembly at an earlier date.

The State Council, acting under the King as president, consists of eleven ministers, of whom the Ministers of the Interior, of Social Service, of Public Instruction, and of Industry have some connection with medical problems.

The political party in power is Socialist. The socialism in the main is one of highly developed co-operation between different sections of the community. Differences of opinion between the two Houses of the Rigsdag have arisen owing, it is stated, to demands on the part of extreme Socialists; but these have not so far been serious.

The chief central offices having control of health and insurance problems are

> The National Board of Health,
> The Board of Social Insurance, and
> The Board for Invalidity Insurance.

To the heads of these three governmental departments I am much indebted for detailed information, though I am alone responsible for any expression of opinion which follows. I should add that in each of these three departments I was much impressed by the activity, enthusiasm, and sound judgment of each of the chiefs concerned. To Dr. Frandsen, the Chief Medical Officer of the National Board of Health, I especially wish to express my obligation.

[1] For further details see *The Statesman's Year Book*, 1929.

The National Board of Health is under the Minister of the Interior, its president being Dr. Frandsen. He, together with the vice-president and a council of expert advisers, supervises the entire public health service of the country, including the whole medical personnel (doctors, dentists, midwives), hospitals, etc., and acts as adviser to the Government in all health matters, medical and hygienic.

A special council under the direction of the president controls the sale of drugs and supervises the whole dispensing system and the personnel.

Further, the medical officers—altogether seventy, mentioned later on—are attached to, and under the direction of, the Board of Health.

To the office of the Board of Health, the administrative work of which is done under the direction of the president, is also attached an expert legal adviser, an expert statistician, and an expert in physics. The last named is concerned with the X-ray installations at the hospitals.

The State Serum Institute is under the Board of Health, and the present director, Dr. Th. Madsen, is adviser to the Board of Health in bacteriology and epidemiology.

A special council, quite independent of the Board of Health and having its own chairman, acts as adviser to the Courts of Justice in legal medical cases.

LOCAL ADMINISTRATION

This is controlled chiefly from the central Government through the National Board of Health. There are 70 district medical officers, of whom 23 act also as county medical officers. In the Faroe Islands there are four additional medical officers, of whom one is the county medical officer.

Corresponding to the 23 county medical officers there are 23 counties, the council of each of these being popularly elected; but its chairman is appointed by the King. The centralised control of appointments will be noted. The 70 medical officers of districts and the county medical officers are appointed by the King on the nomination of the Chief Medical Officer (Dr. Frandsen). They hold office for life and are pensionable. As time goes on, public health matters will probably fall more and more into the hands of the county councils, who will employ whole-time medical officers. The county health officer now supervises the work of district medical officers, holds annual conferences with midwives, and as adviser to the county Epidemic Committee organises uniform control over these diseases.

Outside the 88 boroughs, each with separate local government, administration is through the 23 county councils, with 70 district councils in these counties concerned in local affairs.

So long ago as 1858 it was enacted that each of the 1,400 parishes into which the country is divided should have a local committee of health under the parish council. It is unnecessary to detail the interrelation between these three grades of local authorities, especially as their medical officers are appointed by the Government and are subject to central regulations.

The district medical officers are all part-time officers. Their duty is to treat gratuitously all cases of venereal disease, as well as to advise on health matters.

The district medical officer receives each week a list of all the cases of epidemic sickness which have occurred in the practice of each medical practitioner during the foregoing week. He compiles a summary of these for the county health officer, and sends a monthly statement to the county officer and to the National Board of Health. Although this weekly list must be regarded as somewhat belated for such diseases as diphtheria, informal co-operation is secured immediately in most instances as cases are recognised. Furthermore, immediate notification of certain more serious epidemic diseases to the Board of Health is required.

The district medical officer receives from the parish minister a monthly return of births and deaths, which the

medical officer summarises for his annual report to the
Board of Health. It is part of his duty to superintend to
some extent the work of doctors and pharmacists; and he
must strictly supervise the midwives in his district. He is,
ex officio, a member of the local health committee, and
greatly influences its work. He also carries out legal medical
work in his district, undertaking autopsies as required, and
certifying on mental cases for the police. He is required
also to examine motorists who are suspected of being
intoxicated.

The municipalities and local councils are required to
undertake medical treatment of the poor. In Copenhagen
and a few of the larger towns a special doctor is appointed
for this work, and he receives a fixed salary like any other
municipal officer. In other parts of the country an arrangement is usually made between the local council and one or
more of the general practitioners as to the terms for this
treatment, and the expenses are then defrayed by the
council.

The duty of the medical officer for the sick poor is
usually light, since 66 per cent. of the population on an
average are members of a sickness insurance society.
The general availability of hospital beds also reduces
his work.

The historical importance of the district medical officer
is great. He is a State officer, provided in every district for
treating the poor and for the prevention of disease. In
many parts of the country he is, and has been even more
in the past, the only doctor in the district, though as
prosperity has increased other doctors have appeared. Even
when this is so, the district medical officer occupies still a
privileged position: he is the chief medical adviser in his
district. This historic position, in the view of Dr. Madsen
and other authorities, explains, at least in part, why the
principles of preventive medicine have been so readily
accepted. There is little evidence of friction or controversy
between official and private practitioners of medicine and
between hospitals and private practitioners.

Hospitals

Medical attendance for the poor includes *hospital provision* as well as medical care at home. There is an admirable system of municipal and county hospitals throughout every part of Denmark. Even in its more remote parts a cottage hospital is provided with a complete staff.

At the end of 1924 (*League of Nations' Year Book*, 1925) Denmark had 14,932 beds in general hospitals, including 3,131 beds for epidemic diseases, 889 for diseases of the skin and venereal diseases, and 338 for mental diseases. The total beds for mental diseases in 1928 were 6,953 beds, or 2 per 1,000 of population, most of these in special institutions for the insane. The above total does not include the beds for tuberculous patients—1,321 in sanatoria, 990 in tuberculosis hospitals, and 1,108 in other institutions. There were at the same date 317 establishments for infants, with 5,501 beds.

Charges are made for admission to hospitals, in accordance with the means of the patient. Members of sickness insurance societies never pay personally for hospital maintenance and treatment. For seven-tenths of the total population hospital charges are defrayed by insurance societies, but the amount thus paid only discharges a fraction of the total cost of hospital treatment and maintenance. Thus the charge per patient to insurance societies in a municipal hospital may be only 60 öre a day, while the cost to the municipality will be 10 kroner a day. (100 öre = 1 krone, 18 kroner = £1 or 5 dollars.) Seldom is a payment of more than 2 kroner a day made by the insurance society. The balance of cost comes out of local taxation. There is no indication of objection on the part of taxpayers to support the provision of hospitals and to maintain their professional high standing. Evidently the advantages of high-class hospital treatment are fully appreciated by the general population, and they are willing to pay for this in taxation.

A Local Hospital.—A visit paid to the communal hospital of Aarhus illustrated what I am assured is not a very exceptional quality of hospital provision. Aarhus is a provincial town with a population of about 80,000, and its hospital has 360 beds. At the hospital gratuitous pathological examinations are made for the entire town; and similar provision is made throughout Denmark. The testing for syphilitic infection is undertaken at the State Serum Institute.

Most of the hospital wards have only six beds; some of them are smaller than this. Non-insured patients in these wards pay 4 kroner a day, which covers all charges. Insurance societies' patients are admitted at 2 kroner a day. For a private room 10 kroner a day is charged, and in this case the doctor's fees are additional. The cost to the community of each bed is about 11 to 12 kroner a day. The general provision for patients, including special departments for light treatment, for graduated exercises, for local baths for rheumatism, etc., were admirable.

A tuberculosis block is attached to the hospital, in which 56 patients—observation and febrile cases and advanced cases—are treated. Other tuberculous patients go to the State Sanatorium.

A tuberculosis dispensary is attached to the hospital, in charge of the chief physician of the tuberculosis ward of the hospital. His services are welcomed by other practitioners in the town, the tuberculosis dispensary having been established at their request.

There is no medical inspection of schools in Aarhus. It is pointed out that the inclusion of children in the advantages of sickness insurance renders this less necessary.

The chief physician of the Aarhus hospital is paid 12,000 kroner a year, and he receives also special fees for operations and for patients in private wards.

Dr. Juul, the part-time Medical Officer of Aarhus, to whose kindness I am much indebted, informed me that Aarhus is a port with considerable export trade. It has 67 medical practitioners, including 11 specialists. All the above attend the poor at an agreed tariff, viz. 19 kroner a year for each family.

The relations between Dr. Juul as health officer, the hospital authorities, and the private practitioners of Aarhus impressed me, as also Mr. Kingsbury[1]—who formed the same impression independently—as being extremely satisfactory, all three parties to the medical forces of the community co-operating earnestly and successfully for the common medical good.

HOSPITALS (*continued*)

The hospitals of Denmark have developed to their present advanced position during the last fifty years. In Copenhagen (including Frederiksberg) in 1928 there were 21 hospitals with 7,248 beds, or 10·3 per 1,000 inhabitants. As early as 1806 the King of Denmark—at that time an absolute monarch—issued an Order in Council that each of Denmark's seventeen counties should have one to three hospitals, according to local need. This was very slowly accomplished. As the education of doctors has improved, modern hospitals have been built even in the remoter parts of Denmark. In several counties there is a so-called central hospital, with surgical and medical departments of 100 beds each, attended by specialists. The hospital provision is now mostly modernised, with all known scientific adjuncts. Recourse to hospitals has been greatly increased by charging members of sick benefit clubs not more than half the charge to others. This has been one of the indirect governmental means of encouraging sickness insurance and of securing its present remarkable success in the absence of compulsion by law.

Hospital treatment has also been greatly favoured by the general epidemic regulations, which entitle all infectious patients to free hospital treatment.

It may be said that practically all the surgical work of Denmark, and a very high proportion of its medical work, is done in hospitals. The increasing use of hospital treatment is shown by the fact that in 1901 the number of hospital

[1] Mr. Kingsbury, of the Milbank Memorial Fund, accompanied me in my Scandinavian investigations.

beds per 10,000 inhabitants was 210; in 1919 it had become 260. Most hospitals in the larger centres have special departments for particular diseases. There is nearly always a special section for the treatment of rheumatism.

In Copenhagen there are 16 municipal hospitals and one State hospital. The first named are controlled by a division of the municipal administration, whose chief officer is a director (non-medical).

The 16 municipal hospitals have 5,139 beds, of which 1,673 are for the insane and 129 are in convalescent homes. A Hospital Board is formed, comprising the mayor and an alderman of the city, and the directors of the public health service and of the hospitals service. This Board discusses general hospital problems and arranges the annual hospital budget. A standing committee elected by this Board consists of the hospitals' director and four senior surgeons or physicians; it meets monthly and considers all current hospital problems. The following payments are made for hospital treatment in municipal hospitals by inhabitants of Copenhagen; for non-residents and foreigners the charges are much heavier:—

> In common ward .. .. 1 krone 20 öre per diem
> In single room .. .. 12 kroner per diem

Members of sick clubs are paid for at the rate of 60 öre per diem, and for a member's child only 30 öre during the first 91 days of treatment; after that free treatment is given for a further 13 weeks. Later the patient may become chargeable to the poor law funds.

The charge of 1 krone 20 öre is only equal to about 10 per cent. of the cost of maintenance.[1]

There are, in addition to the above hospitals, other institutions for the chronic sick and disabled and for the old.

The Rigshospital, or University Hospital, in Copenhagen

[1] See article by the hospital directors, K. M. Nielsen and H. F. Ollgaard, *Health Organisation of Denmark,* pp. 309–321.

is a State institution having about 1,000 beds. Patients are
admitted from any part of Denmark. It is the chief centre
for training doctors, midwives, and nurses, and is under
the control of the Minister of Education. Its director is a
jurist, who acts in consultation with the medical council
of the hospital. This council is formed of its senior
physicians and surgeons. Over half of the patients pay
2 kroner per day for treatment; 20 per cent. 4 kroner;
6 per cent. 12 kroner; about 20 per cent. nothing at all.
Of the maternity patients, 70 per cent. pay nothing; the
rest from 2 to 12 kroner a day. Members of those sick
clubs which are authorised by the State pay 2 kroner a
day. The same amount is charged for their children. It
should be noted that, with the exception of the Rigshospital, all general hospitals in Denmark are erected and
supported—so far as the fees charged fail to cover expenses
—by the community to which the hospital belongs and
which has built it. This renders it the more surprising that
the provision is everywhere so liberal and reaches such a
high standard.

It is noteworthy, furthermore, that the large use of
hospitals by persons of all classes appears to be accepted
by private medical practitioners as unobjectionable. There
evidently is behind this position a great weight of irre-
sistible public opinion, apparently concurred in by the
medical profession. This is the more remarkable as hospital
physicians and surgeons are State officers, whole-time or
part-time, living within the hospital grounds and devoting
their chief time to hospital patients, although they may be
allowed facilities for consultations by other patients.

Thus the private doctor partially loses touch with his
patient when the latter enters the hospital, besides losing
fees. He is expected to send notes concerning his patient
on admission; and on the completion of the case the
records are sent to the private doctor for his information.
This interchange is most valuable.

A very high proportion of medical students after
qualifying become residents in hospitals. No doctor is

admitted on the staff of hospitals until he has had exceptional experience in the class of work which he is to undertake.

I asked several doctors whether there was not some risk of over-hospitalisation; and whether it would not be practicable, if adequate home-nursing facilities were provided, to treat many more patients at a less cost in their homes. I was assured that there was no over-hospitalisation, though here and there fear was expressed that the communal burden at present incurred might become excessive. It is evident that the indirect subsidisation of sick benefit societies out of local taxes, constituted by the provision of hospital treatment to the insured at a greatly reduced rate, is a great factor in the demand and the generous provision of hospital treatment. And it is clear that this generous provision of hospital treatment of a high quality has had a great influence in uplifting the standard of medical care for the entire community. It has also an important preventive side, for treatment always implies an educational as well as a curative influence on the patient, and curtailed illness means quicker return to work and a higher standard of health. But has the care lavished on adequate treatment, with the associated fact that district and county medical officers are perhaps devoting more time to clinical medicine and its administration than to preventive medicine, meant a serious loss to public health efficiency? A nearer approach to an opinion on this point will be possible when other sides of medical work have been considered.

MEDICAL ORGANISATION

Active medical practitioners in Denmark numbered in 1928 about 2,500, midwives 1,178, dentists 650, pharmacists 315. Thus there is one doctor to every 1,400 inhabitants. All Danish doctors are trained in Copenhagen, and thus the standard of qualification is uniform. University education is nearly gratuitous, the chief professors concerned in the work being the medical staff of the Rigshospital, aided by the staff of the municipal hospitals of Copenhagen.

The student's training comprises seven years' work.

(1) During the first year of two terms, chemistry, physics, and philosophy (including psychology and logic) must be passed before the student proceeds to—

(2) The study of anatomy, physiology, and physiological chemistry for five terms (two and a half years). During this time the student is required to serve as a "volunteer" every morning in one of the hospitals, in several successive departments. At this stage he learns pathological work, narcosis, and asepsis.

(3) For five further terms the student is engaged in the study of pathology, including bacteriology, pharmacology, and hygiene. He has now reached the end of his sixth year.

(4) In the last two terms (seventh year) he does clinical work only; but similar clinical work is obligatory during period (3) also. Special stress is laid on practical obstetrical work.

About half of the recently qualified men serve a further year's *turnus* service, as assistant in a large hospital.

Nearly all Danish doctors belong to the Danish Medical Association, with the editor of whose chief medical journal, Dr. Kuhn, I had the advantage of discussing Danish medical problems. He was emphatic as to the general good relations between hospitals and sick insurance clubs on the one hand and private practitioners on the other. Sickness insurance had been beneficial in almost abolishing quackery. He did not think that in recent years the increase in incidence of sickness experience found in other countries had occurred in Denmark. As bearing on the almost universal employment of midwives for attendance in child-birth, he did not think that this created difficulty in maintaining the competence of medical practitioners to deal with complicated midwifery. The obstetric education of doctors was thorough; in towns hospitals were always available, and even in rural districts this was so; and district medical officers in remoter parts had ample experience of difficult midwifery.

The Danish Medical Association represents the entire medical profession, and it settles the salaries to be given to hospital doctors, which are liberal, and negotiates with insurance societies as to payment for medical attendance. The Association exerts an important influence on professional conduct, as it can secure the exclusion from insurance practice of any doctor found guilty of unethical conduct. Dr. Kuhn confirmed the statement made by others that in the relation between part-time health officers and other medical practitioners little or no friction was experienced. It appeared to be the universal experience that private practitioners of medicine almost without exception regarded it as part of their duty to help in health matters. The same spirit is manifested in the concurrence of private practitioners in the hospital treatment of such a high proportion of the total cases coming under their care. To the extent to which this co-operation is effective—and it is effective to a remarkable extent—it is a practical expression of that spirit of social service which approaches the ideal formulated by the writer many years ago when "every medical practitioner becomes a medical officer of health within the range of his daily practice".

Nursing

Dr. Frandsen states that there are about 7,000 trained nurses in Denmark. Very largely home nursing has been worked out by special clubs. There are about 800 of these clubs in rural districts, with 900 to 1,000 nurses. Deaconess institutions also provide some 200 trained nurses in towns. In the larger towns municipal nurses tend the poor free of charge. The provision of home nursing on the line of voluntary insurance fits in with the medical insurance arrangements in Denmark.

Midwifery

The practice of midwifery by unqualified women is prohibited. There is one State centre for training midwives, the course of instruction lasting twenty-four months. About thirty midwives are received every year for training. In rural districts the local council are required to appoint as many midwives as are required, the Ministry of Interior deciding the number needed on the advice of the Board of Health. In towns and fairly thickly peopled rural areas these appointments may remain in abeyance when it is proved that there is an adequate supply of midwives engaged in private practice. The supply is not held to be adequate unless at least two midwives are practising in the neighbourhood.

In 1928 there were 697 district midwives. Private practitioner midwives attend women in confinement in all stations in life. A chief Government official informed me that a midwife had attended his wife at the birth of each child, and this appeared to be the general experience. No exceptional difficulty is stated to be experienced in difficult cases, for consultant doctors with special obstetric experience are available in towns, and in rural districts the district medical officer has much experience in difficult midwifery. Most births occur at home. As a rule, only complicated cases are treated in hospitals, with the exception of the Rigshospital for unmarried women and a few private nursing-homes. Not allowing for births in institutions, there is one midwife in Denmark for about 400 births. Some sickness insurance societies pay insured women 2 to 3 kroner a day during ten days after confinement, and may pay for a consultant doctor when needed.

In counties and in cities the health officer confers at least annually with each midwife practising in a given administrative area; and during the year midwives are supervised by the district medical officer.

The local official midwife is provided with a house, is given a salary of 700 to 1,000 kroner, and, in addition, is paid for each case in accordance with the patient's means, the scale being officially specified. She is pensionable, and must retire at the age of seventy. A fourteen days' postgraduate course is offered free. The midwife does her own antenatal work, but must call in a doctor for any abnormality. A nurse as well as a midwife is usually provided, which gives the midwife a higher professional status. The position of the midwife in Denmark is exceptionally strong. Doctors do not concern themselves in private practice with normal midwifery, unless it be to give an anæsthetic. They see complicated cases, but it is understood that a specialist may also be needed.

Poor law regulations in Denmark provide that relief given for the payment of doctors' or midwives' fees or for funeral expenses shall not carry with it the loss of the right to vote in parliamentary and municipal elections, which goes with other forms of poor law relief; and in Copenhagen it has been found necessary for the municipality to guarantee midwives the payment of their fees when the woman in child-birth declares her inability to pay. This includes payment of the midwife for attending on the woman during her removal to the Rigshospital for confinement.

Puerperal Mortality.—In the five years 1925–29 the number of live-births in Denmark was 344,463. The birth-rate in 1922–25 averaged 22·2, and in 1928 had become 19·6, per 1,000 of population; while its infant mortality, 1921–28, varied from 85 to 77 per 1,000 births.

In the years 1925–29 total puerperal mortality in Denmark varied from 2·48 to 3·17 per 1,000 births; in Copenhagen it varied from 2·26 to 3·35 per 1,000 births; and in Frederiksberg, it varied from 2·06 to 5·31 per 1,000 births.

(The joint population of Copenhagen and its suburb, Frederiksberg, is under 700,000, the number of births for Frederiksberg being 55,333 in the five years 1925–29.)

The death-rate per 1,000 births from puerperal sepsis averaged :—

1·05 in Denmark,
1·08 in Copenhagen,
1·30 in Frederiksberg.

(For a general discussion on this subject, see p. 41 and my concluding volume.)

Apart from the experience of Frederiksberg, which is based on rather scanty data, the fact that the experience in

Copenhagen is nearly as favourable as in the rest of Denmark is noteworthy. (Compare pp. 90 and 124.)

CHILD WELFARE WORK

Apart from the valuable work done by district doctors and in hospitals, and the general provision of medical attendance by insurance doctors, there is but little special work in the hygienic instruction of mothers. A similar remark applies to school medical inspection. The Rockefeller Foundation have for a number of years granted the Board of Health some financial help for the establishment of stations for special child welfare work, including the provision of public health nurses working under the local health officer. It is likely that further health nurses will be provided hereafter.

Much special work has been done in providing foster-homes for neglected and illegitimate children, into the details of which it is unnecessary for my purpose to enter.

In 1923 the Child Welfare Act was passed, by which every parish in Denmark was made a child welfare district, and child welfare councils were created. These councils are elected by the parish councils, at least one member being a member of the parish council; the remaining four may be chosen from among residents in the district. In towns the councils are larger. The chief function of these councils is to look after neglected or illegitimate or delinquent children. There are no infant consultations, and domiciliary visits by health nurses are still seldom made.[1]

In Copenhagen eight breast-feeding stations have been maintained for many years, each mother being given a litre of milk daily, subject to her continuance of breast-feeding. Only a very small proportion of mothers attend these stations.

SCHOOL MEDICAL WORK

This work is undertaken on a considerable scale in Copenhagen and a few other towns, but not in the rural districts. The treatment of ailments, except minor con-

[1] See "Child Health in Scandinavia", by Dr. Mason Knox (*Bulletin of American Child Health Association*, November 1928).

ditions, seen to by school nurses, is left to private doctors and to hospitals; and the insurance system renders neglect exceptional.

Tuberculosis Organisation

Denmark has made two outstanding contributions to the prevention and cure of tuberculosis: Bang's method of controlling bovine tuberculosis, and the Finsen light cure of lupus (1895). Great stress is laid on the curative influence of local and general carbon arc-light treatment in tuberculosis, and this is made available in most districts.

Respiratory tuberculosis is notifiable, and special regulations exist limiting the occupation of infectious cases.

The history of tuberculosis is important. In 1890, in towns, the death-rate from total tuberculosis was 3·03 per 1,000, as compared with 2·56 for the whole of England and 2·95 for Sweden. In 1928 the corresponding rates are 0·75 in Denmark (entire country), 0·97 in England, and 1·32 in Sweden. The death-rate from pulmonary tuberculosis in 1928 was 0·55 per 1,000, the lowest in Europe. The fall did not begin until about 1890, since when it has been continuous, excepting a temporary rise in 1917 and 1918. That the decline in tuberculosis has "resulted directly from the measures against this disease"[1] is confirmed by a comparison of the rates of mortality from all causes and from pulmonary tuberculosis in 1876–79, with the corresponding rates in 1900–4 and with 1925–28.

			Total Mortality	Mortality from Pulmonary Tuberculosis
1876–79	..	..	100·0	100·0
1900–04	..	..	78·0	65·1
1925–28	..	..	57·9	28·4

The main provisions made for the control of tuberculosis in Denmark have been the following :—

[1] Report of the Danish National Anti-Tuberculosis Association, 1930.

(1) Every tuberculous patient requiring treatment may be treated in a State-recognised institution, regardless of his ability to pay.

The State furnishes three-fourths of the statutory charge for treatment and care of all patients who cannot themselves pay the full amount. The remaining fourth is paid by the patient himself, or by the sick benefit club, if he belongs to one. In other cases of inability to pay, the municipality pays.

(2) If the breadwinner is in the sanatorium and his family are unable to subsist by their own means, the municipality supplies the family.

(3) The Government gives one-third of the expenses of tuberculosis-stations (dispensaries), and allied arrangements for supervising the hygienic conditions of the homes and families of consumptive patients.

In nine of the twenty-two counties there are tuberculosis dispensaries in which specialist physicians are employed. The tuberculosis dispensaries are largely used by private doctors for consultation and diagnosis. In most districts no friction has arisen; but in some there has been temporary difficulty with private doctors.

There were 16 sanatoria in Denmark in 1928, with accommodation for 1,393 patients. There were also 36 tuberculosis hospitals, with 1,083 beds; and, in addition, 4 invalid homes with 132 beds, 11 seaside sanatoria with 571 beds, 4 seaside hospitals with 428 beds. This gives a total of 71 institutions with 3,607 beds, or 10 beds for every 10,000 inhabitants. There are over 137 beds to every 100 deaths from tuberculosis.

Much importance is attached to the hygienic instruction to patients given while they are being institutionally treated; and great stress is rightly laid on the "epidemiological importance of the patients being removed from their homes in the terminal stages of their disease to such a large extent as is being done" in diminishing the prevalence of the disease. In 1890, in Copenhagen, about 19 per cent. of all deaths from pulmonary tuberculosis occurred in an institution; in 1900 the proportion had become 38 per cent.; in 1912 it was 68 per cent.; and, later, it has become 70 to 75 per cent. Even in rural districts some 30 to 33 per cent. of deaths from pulmonary tuberculosis occur in institutions.

Relief given to the tuberculous patient's family is not regarded as poor relief, and much material help is provided under this heading. The State subsidises the sanatorium or hospital treatment of all patients without means to the extent of 3 kroner per day. This means that at least three-fourths of the total cost of total sanatorium treatment is paid for by the State. The term "without means" is liberally interpreted. Grants in aid are also given for tuberculosis dispensaries.

State aid ceases when the patient returns home, the work then being taken up by the branches of the National Association against tuberculosis in every county. In nearly every district there is a fully-trained nurse who attends the poor free of charge. Sometimes she is an official, more often appointed by an association.

VACCINATION

Vaccination against smallpox has been compulsory in Denmark since 1810. It must be carried out before the child is seven years old, and no child is admitted to school unless it has a certificate of vaccination. Most children are vaccinated at the public expense by the district medical officers; but vaccine is supplied also from the State Serum Institute for private practitioners.

THE TREATMENT OF VENEREAL DISEASES

No feature of Denmark's medical history is more remarkable than its early action against venereal diseases. Free treatment of these diseases had been begun even earlier in some parts of Denmark than in the diocese of Aarhus, which (see also p. 56) was first to have definite regulations, these dating from the year 1788. These prescribed that every person suffering from venereal disease, whether rich or poor, should be given free advice and medicine, and institutional treatment when this was available; that those who failed to report themselves for treatment should be punished; and that the expense of treatment should be borne, not by the parish, but by the whole diocese, consisting of one or more counties. This was, so far as I know, the first instance in which the double duty of the patient to submit to treatment and of the community to treat at its expense was laid down in a legal enactment.[1]

In 1790 the same regulations were put in force throughout Denmark. The free treatment is made part of the official duty of district medical officers, who are not allowed to accept payment for this work. Thus there are seventy doctors in Denmark "part of whose regular duty is the gratuitous treatment of venereal disease". The State pays the municipalities for this. In 1874 the right of everybody, regardless of class or financial circumstances, to treatment at the public expense and the compulsion to submit to treatment were more exactly enacted. In 1906 the police regulation of professional prostitution was abolished, and alternative measures against prostitutes were taken. Of the existent law we need only cite the clause which makes it obligatory on the doctor treating a venereally infected person, when the latter absents himself from treatment, to inform the district medical officer, whose duty is to summon him to resume treatment, if necessary with the assistance of the police. Hospital patients entering to receive treatment at the public expense must not leave without written authorisation from the doctor. All serum tests for syphilis are carried out in the State Serum Institute in Copenhagen free of charge or for a small sum. Dr. Madsen's staff at this Institute made 54,435 tests in 1923; and by means of a card index it is possible to ascertain the exactitude of local returns of syphilis made to district medical officers. The Wasserman test is stated by Dr. G. Tryde to be "used practically always on patients suffering or suspected of suffering from syphilis". He also states that it is made on all the patients in maternity homes. The control of venereal diseases is dependent largely on the experience of medical men in the treatment of these diseases; and it may be noted that every medical student in Denmark is required to go

[1] See Dr. G. Tryde's contribution in *Health Organisation in Denmark*, 1924.

through a three months' clinical course in these diseases, followed by a testing examination.

SICKNESS INSURANCE

Denmark's system of sickness insurance is especially worthy of study. It is unique in that it has become almost universal for those on whom in other countries it has been compulsorily enforced, and yet no direct compulsion has been used in Denmark.

The circumstances leading to voluntary sickness insurance in Denmark resemble those in England. It has been a voluntary growth of personal thrift and mutual helpfulness, which has helped greatly in building up the sense of solidarity in the wage-earning classes or in the members of particular trades. The clubs formed to ensure money benefits and medical attendance in sickness for members and their children, and sometimes provision for funeral expenses, have been worked gratuitously in large measure by members of each club, and municipalities have helped to keep subscriptions at a low level by giving hospital treatment for members at exceptionally favourable terms.

The growth of sick benefit clubs is shown by the following table, giving the proportion per cent. of the total population above fifteen years of age who are members of State-recognised clubs :—

				Per cent.
1893 ..	..	..	..	7·9
1900 ..	..	..	..	18·8
1910 ..	..	..	..	37·0
1920 ..	..	..	..	59·5
1928 ..	..	..	..	65·0

The movement towards growth of voluntary sickness insurance has been greatly aided by the conditions attaching to receipt of aid from the public authorities. The recipient loses his right to vote, he can only marry with the consent of the authorities, and he forfeits his claim to an old age pension if he has received relief during the three preceding years. He is also under obligation to repay relief when he is able to do this. In these ways, and through compulsory insurance against incapacity to work, pressure is brought to bear to secure "voluntary" sickness insurance.

It was not until 1885 that the Government intervened, and then without encroaching on the voluntary character of each club. Sick benefit clubs were given the choice of remaining as they were, or of applying for Government recognition subject to certain conditions and accompanied by special privileges. The obligations were that recognised clubs should comply with certain restrictions of their field of activities and in their account-keeping; a minimum cash benefit was also specified for specified periods in the event of illness. In their turn the Government undertook to subsidise each club on the basis of its membership and subscriptions; to provide payment at very reduced terms in the communal hospitals; and to provide an ambulance at the expense of the municipality to fetch a doctor or midwife for distant patients, or to bring midwifery or other patients to a hospital.[1]

Finally, inspectors were appointed and a Central Board for Sickness Insurance was formed. To Dr. Borgerg, LL.D., the chief official of this Board, and to Mr. Holck, the corresponding head of the Invalidity Insurance Board, as well as to Dr. Frandsen, I am indebted for most of the general information which follows.

A Local Illustration.—As an illustration of the working of a local sickness insurance society, the following example may be given. At Frederikshavn, a small town with a population of 9,900, situated in Jutland, near the most northernly point of the Kattegat, Mr. Kingsbury and I interviewed Mr. Kramer, an assistant master of the local communal school, and by his help also Mr. Andreas Neilson, the secretary of the Familiesygekassen, one of the local sickness associations. There are two further approved societies in Frederikshavn, besides one for railway employees in the provinces of Jutland and Funen. The membership of the Familiesygekassen is confined to the town. Every

[1] Dr. Kuhn's article on the same subject in *Health Organisation in Denmark* is most illuminating.

person is eligible to belong to this Government approved society who has an income of less than 3,800 kroner and a total fortune of 11,700 kroner if single or of 16,800 kroner if he has dependents (according to the tax index of the Board of Assessment), to which 300 kroner is to be added for each child.

Membership is not cancelled strictly when the taxed income[1] increases above these limits. Generally a margin of 20 per cent. is allowed for two or three consecutive years. Then the member is allowed to become a so-called "resting" member. He pays 2 kroner a year, but receives no benefit. If he pays 4 kroner a year he has the right to vote in meetings of the association.

If his income falls to the limit stated above, he again becomes an ordinary member, thus saving the entrance fee of 10 kroner. He may prefer to be transferred to an approved Continuation Sickness Society, whose benefits are about the same, but the contributions to which are 1 krone higher monthly.

The members of the Continuation Sickness Society at Frederikshavn are dispersed over the whole county (Hjorring).

The total membership of the Familiesygekassen, including all members entitled to benefit, comprises 60 per cent. of the population of Frederikshavn. Including the two above-mentioned additional societies, the percentage becomes 75, and including the Railway Association and members of private insurance societies, 96 to 97 per cent. of the entire population are insured.

The business of the Familiesygekassen is done by a committee or governing body of five members, including the secretary. They are elected for two years, two new members being elected every year. The secretary represents the society, presides at meetings, and keeps the list of members. The present secretary has held office for some twenty years. The treasurer keeps accounts, and a collector

[1] The taxed income is the yearly wages declared by the insured person less contributions towards old age pensions and assurances, less also taxes paid in the previous year, and 200 kroner for each child.

is employed to collect the monthly or quarterly subscriptions. The following table shows the money payments and benefits in case of sickness :—

	Payments per Month	Daily Monetary Benefit during Illness
	Kroner	Kroner
A	1.20	—
B	1.50	0.40
C	1.80	1.00
D	2.70	2.00
E	3.50	3.00
F	4.50	4.00
G	5.50	5.00
H	6.50	6.00

Section A applies only to wives, to established workers who receive regular pay during sickness, and to young persons under eighteen. (The master must pay for his apprentices.)

Section B is the largest group.

Section C is the highest group for wives' benefits in ordinary societies.

Section D comprises only twelve members.

If only one parent is insured, an additional payment of 0.25 krone a month is required for children, irrespective of their number. During stay in a hospital only half the monetary benefit is paid.

The monetary benefit for the insured is usually limited to two-thirds of the usual wages, but can be raised to its full amount.

When the benefits and payments are set out in proportional figures (starting with 100 as the base line in each instance), it will be seen that benefits are disproportionately high for those whose weekly contributions are high. (See Figure on page 75.)

It should be stated that only a few benefit from the highest rate of benefit, to which objection has been raised.

The discrepancy between benefits and payments arises from the basic charges incurred by the society.

Doctors under contract are paid a sum which yields 7.20 kroner for each member per year. This covers ordinary professional visits required. The expense incurred by hospital treatment, operations, special visits, daily monetary benefits, and other expenses bring up the expenditure of the society to about 23 kroner yearly per member. It is

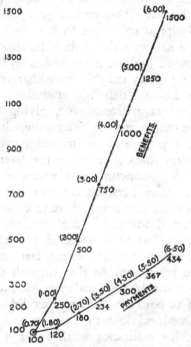

Relation between Sickness Insurance Payments and Benefits.

evident, therefore, that the three lowest rates of payment imply a deficit for the society. The highest rates of payment give an increasing profit.

As most of the members come under the three lowest groups, there is involved in this a deficit of about 27,500 kroner for the society. This deficit is met by subsidies from the Government amounting to about 23,990 kroner and subsidies from the town itself of about 3,000 kroner, with a further small amount accruing from invested savings of the society. These savings have decreased in recent years owing to reductions in public grants.

Of the total contributions from members in 1929, 36,000 kroner were paid to doctors for home treatment and 19,000 kroner to hospitals, of which latter amount 12,300 kroner were paid to the local hospital. In 1930 the hospital expenses are likely to exceed 20,000 kroner. The payment for hospital treatment in the common wards for the insured is 4 kroner a day, half of this being paid by the town. The insured person, if he wishes to be treated in a private room, must pay the difference charged, also half the expense for treatment, including operations.

Six local doctors are employed, giving fair choice of doctors for home treatment. The same doctor must be employed for a year, and an insured person wishing to change his doctor must give notice not later than July 1st in each year. A Reconciliation Committee considers any difficulties that arise between doctors and insured. This committee contains one representative of the society, one of the doctors, and one of the local municipal council.

The doctors appear to be satisfied with their remuneration, and they renewed their contract last year on the same terms as three years ago. At that time all the societies in Jutland thought the doctors' scale was too high and secured a reduction of 10 per cent. The doctors did not strenuously oppose this. One local doctor is stated to earn 18,000 kroner a year out of his insurance work for the local society. The remuneration to the other local insurance doctors averages about 8,000 kroner, one recently settled doctor earning 2,000 kroner from the society.

From the Railway Employees' Society, comprising about 150 members, two doctors earn about 500 kroner quarterly and receive free railway tickets. Two smaller societies comprise 260 and 1,200 members respectively.

From local tax-books the following approximate figures of medical income are derived. They include income derived from private practice. Of course, no such information is obtainable for individual taxpayers.

				Annual Incomes Kroner
Doctors ..	..	..	..	20,000–30,000
Teachers ..	..	..	..	3,400– 5,400
Parsons ..	..	..	..	7,800– 9,000

Average income per inhabitant, 2,085 kroner.

Evidently doctors stand well in the professional scale. In fact, they encourage their patients to join an insurance society, sometimes remitting existing charges if this is done.

It may be added that parliamentary enactment has assisted membership for the poor in these societies. If they cannot pay contributions, these are paid during the first nine months by the Public Assistance or the municipality, and this is not regarded as in the category of poor law relief.

General Remarks on Sickness Insurance.—The sickness funds in Copenhagen have contracts with special doctors. The city is divided into districts, ten to fifteen doctors being employed in each district, from which the insured can choose. Both husband and wife are insured. The doctor is paid 7 or 8 kroner per insured person per annum. No extra charge is made for medical attendance on children under fifteen. The medical charge for man and wife is 14 kroner.

In provincial towns the same system prevails; but in rural districts there is payment for each treatment, in accordance with a detailed tariff. Contracts under each system are made for three to five years, the Association of Sickness Societies and the Danish Medical Association undertaking this task.

Disputes as to these arrangements are stated not to be on a considerable scale, nor is there abuse of the rural system of payment for actual services rendered.

As already indicated, the scale of payment for hospital treatment of insured persons varies within rather wide limits; but the payment never covers more than a part of the expenditure of hospital authorities.

Over-certification of sickness by doctors is not marked. There has been no such phenomenal increase in certification in recent years as has been seen in some other countries.

Unemployment, as elsewhere, does increase sickness certification, but to a minor degree. All the officials interviewed
by me emphasised the high social standard of the Danish
medical profession and their sense of communal responsibility.

About one-fifth of the sickness insurance societies have
contracts with nursing associations for the home nursing
of the insured.

Some societies pay partially for dental treatment of the
insured. There are many women dentists in Denmark.

It has already been stated that most sickness societies
are local, and that there is little overlapping of these
societies. A few societies for railway men, nurses, etc., are
not localised.

Members have the right to transfer to an insurance society
in another locality when they change their abode, and this
right is independent of the member's age or state of health.

Each society has two classes of members, those in good
health when they join, and those who are suffering from a
chronic disease. The accounts of the latter are kept separate,
and the State and municipal authorities jointly pay to each
society the additional cost beyond the average for other
members incurred for the class of invalids.

In Copenhagen there are 70 insurance clubs, but steps
are on foot for large amalgamations. In Copenhagen one
doctor is not allowed to take more than 2,000 insured
persons on his list. The official limit of income for Government grants to insured persons is 4,200 kroner maximum
in Copenhagen, with 300 kroner more for each child. In
smaller towns it varies from 3,800 to 2,800, with an allowance of 300 kroner per child. The Government does not
help the insured with incomes over this limit. There are
said to be some 50,000 insured in this higher class. In these
unhelped middle-class societies the usual arrangement for
medical attendance is that the society allows 4 kroner for
each medical consultation, the patient paying the excess
beyond this if the doctor is not satisfied with the arranged
scale. As already seen, the restrictions of income are not

rigidly adhered to. It need scarcely be added that a person ceasing to be insured cannot recover any payments made by him.

The limits of income include in the approved societies a large proportion of persons who are relatively well-to-do, and, as pointed out by Dr. Kuhn, this has tended greatly to improve the quality and quantity of the services rendered by the societies. But, unfortunately, the subscriptions have tended also to increase, rendering it difficult for the poorest members to remain members.

Whether a remedy will be found for this by making the contributions of the well-to-do heavier than at present in relation to the benefits they receive remains to be seen.

In 1921, according to a table given by Dr. Kuhn, 14·3 per cent. of the total expenditure of over 30 million kroner went in cash benefits, 2·2 per cent. in assistance to women in childbed, 12·9 per cent. in hospital treatment and convalescent homes, 45·4 per cent. in ordinary and specialist medical attendance, and 11·9 per cent. in administration.

The help given by the Government is 2 kroner per member (under the above limitation) per annum; also one-fourth of the expenses of medical or dental treatment and of hospital treatment. In disbursing these contributions the Central Board for Sickness Insurance exercises great control over the finance of local societies. If the experience of a society is unfavourable, a report is asked for as to excessive sickness. One of the two medical inspectors attached to the Board may visit the locality. If the unfavourable experience continues, the society is asked to reduce the benefits given as a condition of the continuance of Government aid. The Central Board of Sickness Insurance as also the corresponding Board of Invalidity are under the Social Welfare Ministry.

INVALIDITY INSURANCE

While sickness insurance is optional, an Act of 1921 provides that all members between the ages of fourteen and forty benefiting by an approved sick benefit club (i.e. having an income below a specified amount) shall be insured against disablement.

Invalidity insurance is a compulsory supplement to voluntary sickness insurance. At the end of 1927 there were 1,425,000 members of sickness benefit societies who were insured against invalidity, i.e. 66 per cent. of the entire population between the ages of fourteen and sixty-two. This compulsory insurance is contributed to by the employer and by the municipality and the State. The compulsory payment of the insured is 5 kroner 40 öre per annum for every person who is insured against sickness before reaching the age of twenty-five, and becomes higher according to age; and the premiums are collected along with the sickness insurance contribution. The employer is required to contribute 5 kroner 40 öre for every worker employed by the year; and these contributions are collected by the insurance societies which are engaged in statutory accident insurance. The remainder of the necessary funds to secure insurance is made up one-half by the State and one-half by the municipalities, the sum thus contributed being allotted in proportion to the number of impecunious members in each municipal area at the end of each year. The benefit accruing on disability consists usually in an annuity of 540 kroner, which in cases of severe invalidity may be increased to 800 kroner by a grant-in-aid from the municipalities, who decide on this on their own initiative. Disability is defined as reduction of working capacity by at least two-thirds.

Evidently the determination of invalidity involves difficult problems which are largely medical. A medical certificate of invalidity may be accepted; but usually collateral evidence from the late employer and others is required. In some instances the local police make inquiries. Often the patient is admitted to a hospital for further observation and report. In 40 per cent. of the total applications a specialist doctor is available. The insurance doctor who first certifies the disability of the insured person is not paid by the Invalidity Board, but he receives 15 kroner from the patient himself.

If the patient can do other work than that in which he was engaged, he remains ineligible for an invalidity pension, as, for instance, a nurse who can do domestic work. If the consultant's written opinion differs from that of the insurance doctor, a copy of it is sent to the latter; and this, it is stated, is usually welcomed.

Measures for the restoration of the health of the invalid are taken when this is possible. This may mean special courses of baths for rheumatism, the administration of insulin in diabetes, and various other measures. Special precautions are adopted to ensure that only annuitants unable to work continue to receive annuities. The heaviest causes leading to invalidity are tuberculosis (14·7 per cent. of the total in 1921–28), diseases of the heart and blood-vessels (9·4 per cent.), chronic intoxications and infections (8·6 per cent.), and a large conglomerate group which is responsible for 26·1 per cent. of the total cases. This includes epilepsy, paralysis agitans, various diseases of the nervous system, insanity, and apoplexy. The last named might perhaps be more suitably placed under circulatory diseases. The chronic intoxications and infections include alcoholism and various forms of rheumatism.

I gathered the impression that regulations as to eligibility for pensions are strict and strictly enforced, and that there is no possibility of political "squeeze" to secure pensions.

OLD AGE PENSIONS

Old age pensions since 1923 are given to persons aged sixty-five without any contributions on the part of the recipients. There is an upper limit of income beyond which these pensions are not given. The present socialistic Government is about to bring in a Bill limiting old age pensions to members of sickness insurance societies. This, along with compulsory invalidity insurance, will go far to ensure that all eligible persons will become insured against sickness.

ANTI-ALCOHOLIC ACTION

In Denmark this problem is greatly agitated, among other reasons, as affecting health insurance and public health.

Many attempts have been made to reduce the consumption of spirits. As in other countries, some degree of control has been found to be essential. Powerful agitation in favour of temperance reform has arisen, and Professor Westergaard states that in some districts the need for this has entirely dominated public opinion. The Great War led to the making of a great national experiment, some details of which are given in my *Story of Modern Preventive Medicine*, 1929 (Williams & Wilkins). Denmark was subjected to blockade, and the Danes had insufficient food. All barley and potatoes were, therefore, diverted from the manufacture of alcoholic drinks, and the price of spirituous drinks was made almost prohibitive. From details given in Dr. M. Hindhede's report, it is evident that, following on the measures taken, deaths from alcoholism and diseases associated with it almost disappeared.

At present stress is laid on high taxation and on limitation of opportunities for obtaining alcohol. Local option is given to municipalities to stop the sale of alcoholic drinks. The municipality can also decide on the number of licensed premises, but they must not exceed 1 to 350 inhabitants.

It is claimed that Denmark in recent years has reduced its consumption of spirits by seven-eighths. The Danes are law-abiding, contented, and prosperous; and police control is effective. As elsewhere, high duties tempt smugglers; but in this respect the national attitude in Denmark—this was the pronouncement made to me by a distinguished Swedish professor—differs from that in Sweden. The Danes, he said, have solved the alcoholic problem by high taxation of spirits, and the Dane will not pay the high price demanded by the bootlegger; while the Swede will maintain that "liquor is always worth its price". The dictum is interesting as a study in national psychology; at the least it emphasises the defensible position that the most efficient law against alcoholic consumption is that which stops short of the point at which it invites the ingenuity and rapacity of the law-breaker to an extent which cannot be repelled.

CHAPTER III

SWEDEN[1]

PRELIMINARY SUMMARY

The medico-social activities of Sweden present features as interesting as those of Denmark. Both countries have a hospital system supported out of taxes, which removes hospital treatment for all needing it from the category of problems still to be solved. At these hospitals patients pay according to their means, but payment to some extent is within the means of the majority of the population.

As is well known, Sweden was the pioneer of official vital statistics, and it now has the longest series of figures giving statistics of marriages, births, and deaths of its population possessed by any community.

As early as 1758 Sweden had an official statistical commission, charged with the tabulation of the returns received from the clergy of each parish, the making of which had become obligatory in 1748. With the initiation of these reforms the names of Elvius, the Secretary of the Swedish Academy of Science, of E. Carleson, and of Per Wargentin will always be associated.

Sweden has adopted the principle of treatment at the public expense of venereal disease in its contagious stages, irrespective of financial status.

In every area of the country is an official doctor, usually appointed by the Government, charged with the medical care of the poor, who can undertake private medical work, subject to an officially fixed tariff, which is very modest.

The majority of women resort to hospitals for childbearing. In municipal hospitals all are attended by fully trained midwives, and at home, nearly all. The training both of midwives and of medical students in midwifery is exceptionally good. The records of puerperal mortality are much lower than in most countries.

[1] Date of investigation, June 1930.

GENERAL OBSERVATIONS

A few general observations are required before considering the points summarised above in further detail.

Sweden, while sharing many characteristics in common with Denmark and Norway, has features peculiar to itself. In 1920 a leading Swedish anthropologist, Carl Fürst, stated that "no people in Europe possess their country with greater home-right than the Swedes". The dolichocephalic, fair, rather tall race seems to be unbroken since prehistoric time in spite of the fact that ancient graves show that a certain crossing with a brachycephalic, dark-skinned race (or several races) has occurred. But as certain dominant racial characteristics—in spite of this crossing during both the Stone and the Iron Age, and, although to a less degree, during prehistoric time—have remained unaltered during thousands of years, the strength of the race is clearly to be seen. It seems to have had a centre of radiation in Central Sweden and Central Norway.

In Denmark the mixture from the southern countries seems to have been greater than in the two other Scandinavian countries.

An element of Fins and Lapps with Mongolian descendants in the north does not even amount to 0·5 per cent. of the whole population.

Sweden can rightly boast of its united character, and of the fact that it has never been under foreign domination. Its people are lovers of winter and summer sports, and they have been the originators of modern systems of physical culture.

The climate of Sweden presents great variations. Sweden has an area half as large again as that of Great Britain and Ireland together. Its greatest length is 1,574 kilometres, its greatest breadth 499 kilometres, and it has an area of 448,440 square kilometres.

In Stockholm daytime in June lasts eighteen hours, and the temperature equals that of Paris in the same month. In winter night is prolonged. More than half the surface of Sweden is covered by trees, which form one of its chief sources of wealth. Next to this in importance comes its valuable iron ore.

The State religion is that of the Lutheran Church. There are two State universities, Uppsala and Lund, and a State faculty of medicine in Stockholm, as well as some smaller private universities. Public elementary education from the age of seven to fourteen is gratuitous and compulsory, and has been so since the year 1842.

The population of Sweden is just over six millions, of whom 40·7 per cent. are engaged in agriculture and fishing, 30 per cent. in industries, and 8·4 per cent. in commerce. Of its total population 69 per cent. live in rural districts.

The general death-rate is about 12 per 1,000, that of Stockholm being only 11 per 1,000. The birth-rate in 1921–25 was 19·4, and in 1928 it was 17·3 per 1,000. Its infant mortality was 62 per 1,000 births in 1928.

GOVERNMENT

Norway seceded from Sweden in 1905. The Swedish King must be a member of the Lutheran Church. Every new law must have his assent, but the right of imposing taxes is vested in the Diet. This Diet or Parliament has two Chambers, both elected by the people. The first or Upper Chamber has 150 members, who are elected on a proportional basis by the members of the county councils (Landstings) and by the electors of the six towns which have separate government from the Landstings. The second or Lower Chamber has 230 members elected for four years by universal bisexual suffrage. The country is divided into twenty-eight constituencies. In each constituency one member is elected for every 230th part of the population of Sweden comprised in the constituency. Every elected member of both Chambers is paid per diem for his services. The Ministry consists of twelve ministers, of whom the Minister for Social Affairs deals with health and medical problems.

Sweden is divided into twenty-five counties, of which Stockholm forms one. One county is divided into two parts, with separate county councils. In Stockholm the head of the administration is a governor, and in the other counties the head is a prefect. The governor and prefects are nominated by the King. They may be said to constitute the supervisory machinery of the Government over local government, and they exercise control over matters of public health in each county. Each county has a medical officer, who advises in professional matters. He acts not only as a medical officer of health, but also as inspector of cottage hospitals and medical institutions. The larger hospitals (*lasarett*), sanatoria, and lunatic asylums are inspected directly by the Royal Medical Board.

The members of each Landsting or county council are elected by the people. Six towns, including Stockholm, Göteborg, and Malmo are administered by their municipal councils separately from county councils.

In addition, every rural parish and every town constitutes a commune or municipality, which deals with scholastic and some other local affairs. They number over 2,500.

Each commune has a council of from three to eleven members elected for four years. They are not paid for their work. In towns special boards are appointed to deal with the services of public health and public assistance, etc. The system of poor law relief does not differ markedly from that of England, except that the communal small units of administration persist. Hospital provision is under separate control from poor law administration.

County Councils are concerned with the wider problems of public health, education and communications. About 60 per cent. of their budget is spent on care of the sick.

MIDWIFERY

In 1925 there were 2,997 midwives in Sweden, as well as 2,116 doctors. According to the *League of Nations' Year Book*, 1,764 of the midwives were attached to districts, while

454 were communal,
  67 were employed in maternity institutions, and
692 were in private practice.

About half the midwives in Sweden are salaried officials. Each of them is supplied with a house. She is allowed to charge fees in addition to her salary. Professor Bovin states that in 1927, 2,895 reporting midwives from the whole country had attended 78,647 confinements, of which 3,481 were miscarriages, and that in over 90 per cent. of these no medical aid had been sought. He gives also the following comparative statement of operative work for the same series of cases :—

	By the Physician	By the Midwife
Manual removal of the placenta ..	712	104
Version	165	18
Forceps	1,393	36
Embryotomy or extraction by hook	72	—

In Stockholm 5,083 births were registered as belonging to the city in 1928, of which 26·5 per cent. were born outside matrimony. As long ago as 1851-60, 43·4 per cent. of the children born alive in Stockholm were illegitimate, and the proportion, though now lower, is still high. This sinister feature is shared by other Scandinavian countries, and by some parts of Germany and Austria. In the maternity institutions of Stockholm the number of births in 1928 was 6,085, of which 5,416 were live-born at term, and 495 were live-born prematurely.

The discrepancy between the figures for the city and for the maternity hospitals arises from the fact that the State hospital admits women from outside Stockholm. Of births in Stockholm only about one-fifth occur in the homes of the people. This movement in favour of institutional treatment is of old standing. It appears likely that ere long there will be few or no home confinements.

At the State Lying-in Hospital in Stockholm (Allmanne Bambordhussett) Professor Forssner[1] courteously explained

[1] A few weeks after my visit Professor Forssner died suddenly. His death removes a distinguished teacher and investigator.

in detail the working of this great institution, of which he is the head. It is an old foundation, dating from the year 1775. Some 3,500 normal deliveries take place in it yearly, not including abnormal cases and abortions. The hospital has a separate gynæcological section. In the municipal hospital, which is more centrally situate in Stockholm, nearly the same number of deliveries occur. Medical students are trained in the State hospital, and midwives in the municipal hospital. The State hospital has attached to it a polyclinic or out-patient department, at which about 5,000 women attend yearly. Some of these are gynæcological cases. Many patients attend to ascertain if they are pregnant, and attendance at the polyclinic from the fifth or sixth month of pregnancy is common. Cases of eclampsia are few, and Professor Forssner informed me that among these the case mortality does not exceed 5 per cent.

Intentional abortion appears to be common; a fact which fits in with the high illegitimacy rate. As doctors must not produce abortion except for serious illness, patients who have been to charlatans often come to this hospital for septic complications. There is a special operating-room for infected cases. All patients showing fever are isolated in a special department. Premature births are also relegated to a special department. Special nurses are employed, and one or more wet-nurses.

Institutional midwifery is increasing to such an extent as to render it likely that ere long there will be but little need of domestic midwifery.

The Training of Doctors in Midwifery covers a period of four months, during which every medical student in Stockholm[1] must reside in the State Lying-in Hospital, two months as a junior and two months as a senior. There are always twenty-five students in the hospital. During his first two months the junior must always accompany a senior student, undertaking under the latter's supervision whatever would otherwise be done by a midwife. Vaginal examinations are allowed for educational purposes. There are no

---

[1] The same arrangements hold in Uppsala and Lund.

midwives at this hospital. During his senior period the student takes the place of a midwife, and undertakes all her work. He will have from forty to fifty normal deliveries at full term and from eight to ten miscarriages, and will probably have two or three forceps cases. He helps in other operations. Cæsarean section is not uncommon, although rickets is exceptional. It may be necessitated by placenta prævia, uterine inertia, etc. The medical students are trained in aseptic methods, including the washing of hands with water and then spirit, followed by the use of gloves. Midwives must use antiseptics.

The patients at the State hospital mostly pay 2·5 kroner (about 2s. 10d., or 60 cents) a day for eight days, if treated in the general wards; more in private wards. After the eighth day, if the patient needs to be retained, no charge is made in the general wards. The municipality of Stockholm and the State share between them the residual cost of the State hospital above the charges paid by patients. In the town hospital the municipality pays this excess of cost. A like system holds good in all towns throughout Sweden, also in most of the Swedish counties.

Hospital delivery has done much to reduce sepsis in parturition. In the statistics given below deaths from septic abortion are included.

The Training of Midwives is carried out in two Government schools, in each of which fifty to sixty students are resident. Since 1924 the course of training lasts two years; before that it was one year. Now also two post-graduate courses of a fortnight are obligatory before the midwife is fifty years old. She has to retire at the age of fifty-five. If a midwife has had much experience with a district doctor, she can be exempted from the review courses by the doctor's certificate. Midwives are allowed to do certain operations in rural practice if a doctor is unavailable. Professor Bovin shows that this permission is imperative, especially in northern districts, in which the population may be only two or three to every square kilometre. A doctor may be unavailable, and the midwife must therefore be taught manual removal of retained placenta, external and internal version, extraction in breech presentations, and even the use of the low forceps. During her training each student has the opportunity to conduct eighty to one hundred deliveries. She also receives training in a pediatric clinic.

Apart from the exceptional circumstances indicated above, the midwife must call in a doctor when complications occur.

Professor Forssner confirmed the general Scandinavian experience that no serious consequences accrue from doctors not ordinarily attending confinements. The training of medical students in obstetrics is very thorough; in towns specialists are available as well as hospital treatment; and in rural districts doctors continue their experience of complicated midwifery.

Sweden has a remarkably low mortality from complications due to pregnancy and parturition. This is only about 2·5 per 1,000 live-births, as compared with 4·5 in England, and with a still higher rate in America. There appears to be no doubt that the difference cannot be explained, except possibly to a small extent, by variations in completeness of certification of causes of death.

In Stockholm, judging by the statistics of the five years 1924–28, extracted by me from the annual statistical report of the city, and kindly confirmed by the city statistician, Dr. J. Guinchard, the puerperal death-rate is higher than that in England and Wales as a whole, which was 4·42 per 1,000 births in 1928, as compared with 4·88 in Stockholm.

The table on the facing page shows the exact figures for Stockholm.

Assuming the accuracy of the figures for Sweden as a whole, is the much higher proportion of deaths from sepsis in Stockholm the result partially of purposeful abortions; or can it in part be due to the additional risks associated with the training of medical students and midwives?

If the lower figure for Sweden as a whole be accepted, it can properly be ascribed to the high quality of the training of both doctors and midwives, to the high proportion of institutional confinements, and to the high standard of

cleanliness of the people as well as of their attendants. The
uniform as well as the high standard of training must be
remembered, and the fact that antisepticism or asepticism
is rigidly enforced. Systematised antenatal work does not
appear to have borne a considerable part in securing the
low puerperal mortality.

FIVE YEARS, 1924–28

	Stockholm	All Towns of Sweden
Total births	26,008	
Deaths from puerperal sepsis	93	191
Deaths from eclampsia	11	
Deaths from other complications of pregnancy and parturition	23	163
Total	127	354

CHILD WELFARE WORK

The fact that elementary education of children has been
compulsory and gratuitous since 1842 implies a degree of
intellectual enlightenment highly conducive to advanced
measures for the prevention and treatment of disease. As
long ago as 1624 it had been enacted that material assistance
given to children should be separated from that given to
others, and that special asylums for them should be created.
It is unnecessary to describe the various institutions and
agencies now concerned in this work, as they bear only
indirectly on medicine. Every commune is required to form
a child welfare board, one of whose duties is to care for
foster-children.

Formerly there were many *gouttes de lait*. These are now
largely replaced by infant consultations in many areas; but
the latter are not found in all areas, and there is no general
organisation corresponding to the systematic home visita-

tion of mothers and their infants in Great Britain, made by nurses specially trained in this hygienic work. In Stockholm the municipality give premiums to mothers while nursing their infants. In 1928 the help thus given amounted to 60,596 kroner (about £3,460); and during the same year 1,962 boarded-out infants were under municipal surveillance.

School Medical Work

This work is not very fully developed outside Stockholm and a few towns. It is claimed that the abundance of available hospital treatment renders school medical work somewhat less necessary.

In the treatment of dental diseases there has been much activity. As seen on page 98, over 26,000 children attending primary schools received dental care at polyclinics, out of the total 30,000 scholars attending school, at a cost of about 300,000 kroner.[1] In about half the Swedish towns and in some other districts there are school dental clinics, at which gratuitous dental treatment is given. The growth of dentistry in Sweden has been rapid. In 1854 there were only fifteen qualified dentists. In 1897 a school for the training of dentists was started, and in 1928 there were 933 qualified dentists practising in Sweden.

The Hospital System

The hospital system bears a general resemblance to that of Denmark. It is national in character, the expenditure being borne chiefly by taxation and the payments of individual patients.

In 1927[2] there were—

18,085 beds in county and cottage hospitals, including obstetrical beds,
6,309 beds in sanatoria and cottage hospitals,
6,962 beds in fever hospitals, and
12,118 beds in mental hospitals,

[1] L'Œuvre Sociale en Suède (Government Publication, Stockholm, 1928).
[2] The Official Hospital Organisation in Sweden, Nr. 59, p. 30 (Publication of State Medical Board).

altogether between 43,000 and 44,000 beds; while private hospitals provided 3,303 beds.

The extent to which the total running expenses of all the above institutions was borne by patients' payments may be seen below:—

Total running cost of general hospitals, including   Kroner [1]
   the first three groups named above   49,892,000
Total running cost of mental hospitals   18,114,000

   Percentage proportion of cost borne by:—

	General Hospitals	Mental Hospitals
Contributions from patients	29·8	38·6
Donations	1·9	nil
State contributions	9·8	61·4
State or communal contributions ..	58·5	nil
Total	100·0	100·0

The State makes itself responsible for mental hospital accommodation, the administration of these institutions being directed by the State Medical Board of the Central Ministry. Additional beds have been provided by the county councils, because of deficiency of State provisions.

The communes or districts, although primarily responsible for care of the destitute, leave the provision of most of the institutional accommodation needed to the county councils, except for a certain number of chronic and incurable cases. Even this is likely to be transferred to the county councils. During the last decade the Board of Pensions, which is in charge of old age and invalidity pensions, has opened up a third source of hospital provision. This has been especially for chronic rheumatism, neuroses, and after-consequences of accidents etc., with a view to minimising the prolonged invalidity apt to be produced by them. In recent years there has been increased provision

[1] 1,000 Swedish kroner = 268 dollars.

by the Board of Pensions of a special department for rheumatism in general hospitals. There are now five such hospitals with 260 beds.

The transport of the sick is largely provided by public contributions. The Red Cross organisation has taken an important part in this work, including the enterprising provision of aeroplane ambulances in some remote northern districts.

The progress made in hospital provision is shown by its doubling between 1907 and 1927, or, more accurately, its increase from 3·7 beds to 8·1 beds per 1,000 inhabitants.

As already indicated, the twenty-five county councils of Sweden and the municipalities of its six largest towns provide the hospital accommodation for the people, except its mental hospitals, for which the State is responsible; although in this case also some supplementary beds are provided out of local funds. The local hospitals are called "lasaretts" if more than thirty beds are provided, and cottage hospitals if less than this number. At the end of 1927 there were 93 general hospitals, with 16,847 beds, and 74 cottage hospitals, with 1,238 beds.

In all counties, except five, the hospitals are already divided into a surgical and a medical department and an X-ray department. Nearly all the counties will, before long, have at least one hospital at their disposal which is divided in this way. In some counties there are also departments for ear, nose, and throat sicknesses, and provisions for maternity cases. A State committee is at present considering the question of medical attendance, and a more detailed plan is being made for the division of the hospitals into special departments.

In the largest cities there are separate maternity hospitals. In 1927 there were 827 beds for this purpose in special or general hospitals.

In Lund there is a hospital with 728 beds, and in Uppsala a hospital with 585 beds, which receive large State subsidies, as well as county contributions, in aid of clinical education. Karolinska Institut in Stockholm, which provides for training of doctors, like that given at the Universities of Lund and Uppsala, has attached to it the Serafinerlasarettet with 452 beds, as well as several wards in the municipal hospitals of the capital, for clinical tuition. These hospitals are admirable in their arrangements, and well repay a visit.

The administration of hospitals and sanatoria for tuberculosis is regulated by Act of Parliament. A Board of Governors is appointed by the county council for each general hospital, one of the medical officers of the hospital acting as its superintendent and reporting to this Board. This superintendent is appointed by the Government.

The State Medical Board sends inspectors to the various hospitals, and its approval is necessary for all new hospitals or the enlargement of hospitals. The medical officers of cottage hospitals are appointed by their governors.

The fees chargeable to patients are decided by the county council, and they vary in different localities. For residents the average fee is 1 krone 75 öre a day (nearly 2s., or 50 cents), but it may be as high as 5 kroner for persons of economic competence. In rooms with 2 to 4 beds the payment is 4 to 6 kroner, and in single rooms may be 7 to 10 kroner. These charges include all nursing and medical expenses.

The doctor has not the right to receive remuneration from a patient who has been taken care of in a public ward. An advisory rate of doctors' fees from patients in private and half-private wards has been issued by the State Medical Board. Except in a few hospitals, patients are under no obligation to remunerate the doctor who has taken care of them in general hospitals.

Stockholm has numerous hospitals coming under three headings (see tables on following page).

At these hospitals charges are made, except for the indigent. At the Sabbatsberg Hospital 2 kroner 50 öre is the charge per day for inhabitants, and 8 kroner for outsiders. Nurses and public health nurses are trained at this hospital. There are surgical, medical, and special departments, and the medical head of each of these has also private practice, but the assistant doctors, as a rule, have not. From 11.30 to noon out-patients at the eye department were received at a charge of 2 kroner. Later in the day the doctor can see patients

A. UNDER THE MUNICIPAL COMMISSION OF HEALTH, 1928

	Number of Beds	Number of Patients Admitted
Sabbatsberg Hospital	728	10,839
St. Goran Hospital	593	2,062
Aso Hospital	102	901
Katarina Hospital	11	161
Maria Hospital	241	4,260
St. Erik Hospital (Section for Bodily Disease)	1,009	3,954
Municipal Maternity Hospital	111	3,585
Epidemic Hospital	616	2,060
Soderby Hospital	444	949
Hamra Sanatorium for Infants	37	63
Tjarnan Sanatorium for Infants ..	100	101
S. & M. Sachs Hospital for Infants ..	46	361
Langbro Hospital for Insane	820	487
St. Erik Hospital (Section for Insane) .	387	76
Other Hospitals for Insane	508	174
Total of A	5,753	30,033

B. UNDER THE MUNICIPAL COMMISSION OF PUBLIC ASSISTANCE, 1928

Högalid Hospital	328	576
Eira Hospital for Venereal Diseases ..	100	539
A and B	6,181	31,118

C. OTHER HOSPITALS, INCLUDING SOME PRIVATE HOMES

	2,067	25,975

at the hospital and can charge up to 10 kroner, but 1 krone must be given to the hospital. In other departments the surgeon does not receive payment from out-patients. The system is not without disadvantage to the patients. There is, as in the out-patient departments of English hospitals, often prolonged waiting before the patient is seen.

POLYCLINICS

The above is part of the system of polyclinics initiated in recent years by the municipality of Stockholm. Mostly these polyclinics are intended for general medical cases. Patients are allowed to come to these polyclinics without reference from a private doctor. They pay 2 kroner for each consultation. Evidently this must encroach on private medical practice. At some of the clinics connected with the educational clinics in Stockholm hospital the treatment is free of charge in many cases.

I was informed that at Uppsala the opening of a polyclinic a few years ago had been strongly opposed by the local doctors. It was asserted that many patients, even when sent by the private doctor for expert advice, did not return to him, notwithstanding the rule of sending patients back to doctors who have referred them to a polyclinic for an expert opinion.

Apart from the polyclinics at the University hospitals in Uppsala and Lund and the large public hospital in Göteborg, polyclinics are not situate at the hospitals; but the chief physicians at these hospitals, with the permission of the governors, have their private practice in the hospitals, and in their absence the assistants also treat patients who do not need to be admitted as in-patients. The fee for these treatments is generally low. The physicians at some hospitals pay for the X-ray plates and for assistance required at these hospital clinics.

The reception of patients at the polyclinics independently of family doctors means much loss of private medical practice. I was informed that here and there outside of towns there was little private practice; and that in towns the chief obstacle to the overwhelming success of polyclinics arose from the long waiting of patients. Many patients rather than suffer this go to private doctors.

The extent of activity of the polyclinics in Stockholm—

which are either municipal or are subsidised by the municipality—will be seen below. The figures relate to the year
1928 and to Stockholm alone.

1928
Number of Persons
cared for

At Municipal Polyclinics 114,250
At Subsidised Polyclinics 80,429

Population of Stockholm 474,094

The patients treated at polyclinics were distributed as
follows :—

A. MUNICIPAL

Sabbatsberg Hospital	46,820
St. Göran Hospital	7,689
Maria Hospital	15,233
St. Erik Hospital	1,044
Sach Infants' Hospital	1,215
Polyclinic at Södermalm	5,730
Other Polyclinics	9,980
Polyclinics for Primary Schools	26,539
	114,250

B. SUBSIDISED POLYCLINICS

Polyclinic at Ostermalm	2,059
Seraphins Hospital	48,679
Deaconesses' Hospital	2,692
Princess Louise Hospital for Sick Children ..	4,950
Carolin Institute for Infants	4,775
Dental Institute	12,298
Polyclinic for the Deformed	1,766
Radium Institute	3,210
	80,429

The above tables do not completely state the multiplicity
of arrangements for expert consultation at various hospitals
or at polyclinics independent of hospitals. Commonly one
hospital has several polyclinics. Thus, at the Sabbatsberg
Hospital there are special clinics for medical, surgical,
gynæcological, and ophthalmic cases, and for diseases of
the ear, nose, and throat.

St. Goran's Hospital has special polyclinics for skin,
urinary, and venereal cases, and for phototherapeutics.

SICKNESS INSURANCE

Sickness insurance in Sweden, as in Denmark, is on voluntary lines; but it has not developed in Sweden to the same extent as in Denmark, in which country it has become almost a religious duty to insure. Accident insurance was first in the field. In 1901 an Act was passed by the Swedish Diet indemnifying workers for accidents occurring while at work; and this came into operation in 1903. This did not apply to agricultural and transport workers, or to maritime occupations. In 1915–16 the Act was made more generally applicable, the employer paying the premium for insurance. Certain industrial diseases are now included in the insurance. The employer must insure his employees against accident. He can do this through a private company. If he does not do this he comes automatically under the State Accident insurance system. The law provides for reduction of the insurance premium for employments in which accidents do not occur. Four engineers are attached to the State Insurance Office against Accident to advise as to the prevention of accidents. I am indebted to the General Director of this office, Mr. Sigurd Ribbing, for valuable information on this branch of work. When an accident has been due to serious imprudence or to the drunkenness of the worker, the indemnity can be reduced, after a judicial inquiry, to a reasonable extent. An attempt is being made to introduce the alcoholic blood-test for police cases. In the last few years there has been a marked increase in claims for compensation for accidents. In the first four months of 1930 there was an increase of 30 per cent., as compared with the same months in 1929.

Several reasons are given for this. Rationalisation means an increase in the pace at which work is done; the introduction of more "piecework" has had the same effect; and workers apply to a larger extent for minor accidents than formerly.

Sick clubs have long existed in Sweden, as in other northern countries. Increase of industrial life in Sweden gave an impetus to these clubs. In 1910 the present legislation was introduced which, while it left the initiative to private societies to insure contributors on voluntary lines, provided for granting subsidies, under certain conditions, from the national Treasury, in aid of the benefits offered by these societies. These benefits usually covered sickness, maternity, and funeral expenses. After inquiry, the Government in 1926 still favoured voluntary sickness insurance. The State supervises societies which are registered. These are subject to certain regulations as to finance and general management, this work being entrusted to the Department of Labour and Social Welfare (Socialstyrelsen). In 1928 there were 1,223 registered societies in Sweden, with 912,919 members. If unregistered societies be included, one-fifth of the adult Swedish population belongs to a sick club.

In 1924 the number of societies was 1,264, of which 462 were local urban funds, 770 were local rural funds, 32 were national funds.[1]

The vast majority of members belong to miscellaneous local societies; only a small minority belong to Trades Union Funds, Works Funds, and Occupational Funds.

Invalidity due to old age is not regarded as sickness in the administration of the societies. The amount and duration of sickness benefit and the premiums payable by the insured vary greatly in different societies. Commonly the insured person pays about 22 kroner per annum.

The State subsidy at first was limited to helping in the administration of the sickness societies. After the Act of 1910 subsidies were increased, and in 1921 included the following items[2]:—

(1) 2.00 kroner per member per annum.
(2) 25 öre (one-fourth of a kroner) for each day of incapacity, excluding Sundays, during which the society has paid during the preceding year at least 90 öre, or has maintained the patient in a hospital.
(3) An allowance of one-fourth of the cost of medical and

[1] *Voluntary Sickness Insurance*, International Labour Office, Geneva, 1927.
[2] This list is incomplete. For further details see *loc. cit.*, p. 377.

pharmaceutical expenditure for insured persons during the preceding year, subject to a maximum limitation.

(4) When maternity is the subject of insurance, and the sickness society pays for not less than fourteen days either 90 öre a day, or bears the expense of the insured in a maternity home, and when the patient also is insured against sickness, the Government pays 60 öre for each day during which the society has paid maternity benefit.

The Act of 1910 does not provide for communal subsidies. These are entirely optional on the part of communal authorities; so likewise are contributions from employers. The amount of these in 1927 is seen below:—

Registered Societies

	Kroner
Contributions received from the insured:	
Regular contributions	18,566,196
Supplemental contributions	336,967
Contributions received from employers	291,177
Contributions received from the State (regular)	3,307,694
Contributions received from the State (supplemental)	89,821
Contributions received from the Communes	505,629

It should be added that legally there is no limitation of income for sickness insurance, and that any person thus insured is entitled to the full benefits given in virtue of his contributions.

No outstanding difficulty appears to have been experienced in the relation between private and medical practitioners and the sick clubs. Medical attendance is given only in a few clubs; most clubs pay only a monetary benefit, the insured paying for his own medical certificates. Doctors employed by insured persons are commonly paid by fee per attendance. In cities special doctors are sometimes employed. Commonly also the insured person pays for his own hospital treatment.

At the present time (May 1930) social provision in Sweden is characterised by a great lack of co-ordination between its different schemes—provisions for accidents, sickness insurance, and old age pensions—and, in consequence, unnecessary complications of administrative machinery. The need for a more rational organisation is also growing more and more pronounced. In conversations objection was occasionally expressed to the introduction of compulsion for sickness insurance, the view taken being that insurance once it becomes compulsory loses its character and becomes a system of taxation.

ORGANISATION OF THE MEDICAL PROFESSION

A large part of the medical profession in Sweden is employed in the service of the State, most of these not as full-time officials. There are 2,200 doctors in Sweden, or about 1 to 2,900 persons.

On its public health side, medicine is well represented in the Central Service of the State, with Dr. Nils Hellstrom as its chief medical director. To him I wish to express my obligation for valuable help, as well as to Mr. Huss, the General Director of Social Services, to Mr. Ribbing at the head of the department dealing with State contributions to social insurance, and to Mr. von Koch, chief of the department of poor relief.

Dr. Hellstrom's department is concerned not merely with the problems of public health in the stricter sense, but also with domiciliary and pharmaceutical medical practice and hospital practice throughout Sweden, including the control of mental asylums and of anti-tuberculosis institutions.

The whole country is divided into so-called provincial physicians' districts, and in each of these districts a doctor appointed by the Government and paid by the State has his station. It is his duty to give medical attendance to the inhabitants in his district for fees fixed by the Government. The communities have to pay the fees of the poor to the provincial doctors. In a *few* districts these provincial doctors are appointed by a local board and paid by this board with contributions of the State and the county council. In the cities there are several district doctors, or "city doctors", whose duty it is to give the poor free medical attendance. These doctors are appointed by the city council. These "city doctors" are not bound by any special fee for their private practice. In every town one doctor has the duties of a health officer.

I am assured that there is no evidence of neglect of the poor when the doctor's private practice increases. Each commune is under legal obligation to give monetary and medical aid to the destitute; and the prefect of the county has power to compel this, if there is local neglect. In cities there are several district doctors for the poor paid by salaries. They are allowed to undertake also private practice; but throughout Sweden the fees charged in this private practice must be in accordance with a tariff laid down by the Government, so far as the local inhabitants are concerned. Others may be charged higher fees. This limited tariff for private patients is not enforced in Stockholm. In country districts the tariff has had a marked influence on the fees chargeable in private practice.

Each county has a whole-time chief medical officer. His duty is to supervise the general hygiene in the county, to inspect cottage hospitals, sick homes (homes for chronic diseases), poor-houses, children's homes, and similar institutions for general welfare. It is also his duty to inspect the official activities of the provincial doctors, but not their private practice work. His appointment is permanent, and he is a pensionable officer. The central control of poor relief exercises a more general supervision of this work, nine assistant inspectors being engaged in this duty.

In Stockholm and Göteborg there are two medical officers of health appointed by the State and the Municipality. In addition, there are assistant doctors who combine public health and medical attendance on the poor. Stockholm is subdivided into nineteen districts, in each of which is a district doctor whose duty it is to give medical attendance to the indigent. The number of sick persons thus attended in 1928 was 11,794, or 2·5 per cent. of its total population. Of those attended about 17 per cent. were removed to hospital.

The city M.O.H.[1] is at the head of the hospital depart-

[1] M.O.H. means Medical Officer of Health.

ment of the city. There are twelve municipal hospitals, and eight others which receive contributions from the city funds.

Reference is made on page 97 to the city polyclinics, which appear to function in almost direct competition with private practitioners, and not solely as consultation centres.

In Stockholm fifteen nurses are employed for domiciliary nursing of the poor. The large amount of hospital treatment reduces the need for these. Outside the cities there are district nurses, half of whose salaries are paid by the commune and half by the Government.

VENEREAL DISEASES

The control of venereal disease in Sweden does not include the inspection of prostitutes, which ceased in 1910. A Commission sat on revised regulations from 1903 to 1910, and in 1918 Parliament adopted the medical proposals made by Dr. Marcus and his colleagues on the Commission.

(1) A definition of syphilis in an infectious stage was adopted. This denoted a case of this disease during the first three years after infection; and for women a positive Wassermann up to the menopause.

(2) The duty was imposed on every patient to seek medical advice, which from that time was made gratuitous. Previously free treatment could only be obtained in large towns and in the University clinics. Now every town with a population of more than 20,000 has polyclinics to which specialists are attached. In smaller towns and in rural districts free treatment is given by the district medical officers. The arrangements provide for a fixed tariff to the doctors attached to the polyclinics and to the district medical officers. All fees are paid by the State, except salaries of nurses and rent of rooms, which are provided by the local commune.

(3) As a correlative to free treatment, the patient is under the obligation to pursue his treatment. If he does not do so, the method adopted is shown below:—

Notice in accordance with the Official Law of 1918, sent privately from the doctor to the patient.

Name...................Occupation...................Address...............

Inasmuch as you have, contrary to par. 9 of the above law directed to preventing the spread of the infection of venereal disease, discontinued treatment by me, without proof that treatment has been taken over by another doctor, you are instructed to come to see me before.....................(date) or to prove that treatment is now being carried on by another doctor. Failing this the matter will be reported to the health inspector of the municipality.

> Signed (Name of doctor).
> Date.................Address.......................
> Hours of Attendance.......................

If this notice is not complied with, the clinician is required to send the following notice to the health inspector of the district:—

Notice according to par. 9, etc., to the Medical Health Inspector.............................

[Here follows name, year of birth, civil status, occupation, and home address of the patient.]

whom I have treated for.............................has neglected to abide by my instructions, inasmuch as.. .....has discontinued treatment with me without proving to me that treatment has been taken over by another doctor.

> Remarks...

The health inspector then writes to the patient; and if he then does not resume treatment, the police are informed. If after two admonitions by them the patient still does not return for treatment, they are authorised to conduct him to the clinic. This is very seldom required.

Dr. Marcus informed me that during the last ten years there has been little failure to complete treatment. There are three public clinics for venereal diseases in Stockholm. At Dr. Marcus' clinic at St. Goran's Hospital every day about 120 men and 150 women are seen for venereal and skin diseases. The staff consists of three doctors, who are assisted by medical students. The staff is salaried, no payments by patients being allowed.

(4) The physician in charge of the venereal disease clinic is expected to ask every patient as to the source of infection, and the physician is required to report to the health inspector if he regards a probable source of infection as established. The health inspector then writes to the suspected person, making an anonymous statement and advising recourse to a doctor within two or three days. The suspected person is further asked to report the result of this examination. This machinery was discussed for several years, jointly by doctors and lawyers; and the conclusion reached by the doctors was that, while aware

of the importance of maintaining medical secrecy, this case justified exceptional treatment. In 60 per cent. of a large series of cases the source of infection was traced.

(5) Every doctor is required to make a statistical notification of each case of venereal disease, and of its supposed source of infection, on the same day as he has seen his patient. No fee attaches to this.

The arrangements for the treatment of venereal disease at Dr. Marcus' clinic at the St. Goran Hospital were admirable.

The statistics of notified cases show considerable reduction of venereal disease in Stockholm. The following table from a contribution by Dr. Marcus, 1928, shows, if we may assume that the figures are fairly comparable, that venereal disease is diminishing in Stockholm and in Copenhagen, but increasing in Oslo. The figures relate to all forms of venereal disease in the aggregate.

AVERAGE NUMBER OF CASES OF VENEREAL DISEASE PER 1,000 INHABITANTS IN THE YEARS—

	1913 and 1914	1925 and 1926
Stockholm	18·9	10·7
Copenhagen .. (Denmark)	18·3	13·6
Oslo (Norway) ..	8·4	11·6

The compulsory notification of venereal diseases renders possible a comparison of the known cases of syphilis and gonorrhœa from the year 1918, when the present methods of control became obligatory.

No. OF CASES IN EACH YEAR OF—

Year	Syphilis	Gonorrhœa
1919	5,823	20,471
1920	3,221	14,996
1926	912	12,610
1927	1,168	12,439

There is stated to be very little venereal disease in rural districts. Private doctors make no objection to the venereal polyclinics. The publicity attaching to these is stated to lead remunerative patients to come to the private doctors instead of to the clinic.

Furthermore, the practitioners in Sweden, as in Denmark, have been so long accustomed to the institutional treatment of disease, partially at the expense of taxes, that it is accepted as part of the natural order of things.

Dr. Marcus, the distinguished syphilographer, to whom I am indebted for much of the above information, is also in medical charge of the Welander Home, situate close to the St. Goran Hospital in Stockholm. This home is one of three in Sweden; and other homes of a similar type have been opened in Denmark and Norway. It is intended for young children suffering from congenital syphilis between early infancy and the age of four to five years, or a little higher. The first homes of this kind were initiated by the late Dr. Welander, of Stockholm, thirty years ago. He pointed out that to cure congenital syphilis in children early intensive treatment and continuous care are required.

In this institution some fifty children are treated under admirable conditions. One could not fail to be impressed with the homelike character of the institution and the beneficent work it evidently accomplishes.

The statistics of Sweden confirm the conclusion that congenital syphilis has declined greatly.

It will be seen that the three points in the Swedish system for the control of venereal diseases are: (1) free treatment for all applicants, (2) obligation on the part of the patient to complete his treatment, and (3) vigorous efforts to trace the source of infection in each case. Attempts at the personal sanitation of prostitutes by periodical examination have been abandoned; but heavy penalties attach to the transmission of disease.

TUBERCULOSIS

There are over two hundred tuberculosis dispensaries in Sweden, which are supported by the county or communal councils, aided by subsidies from the State. In addition, there are many institutions for the residential treatment of tuberculosis. In 1897 the Swedish people subscribed 2,200,000 kroner as a gift to King Oscar II on the twenty-fifth anniversary of his reign, and he gave this for the building of sanatoria. Further money was contributed by the Diet, and with the sum thus secured four sanatoria were opened, with 508 beds in all, for the treatment of early cases of tuberculosis. At the end of 1928 the accommodation provided was as follows:—

	Beds
At 33 Sanatoria	5,015
„ 52 Cottage Hospitals for tuberculosis	1,179
„ 13 departments in general hospitals	733
„ 5 seaside sanatoria	1,144
„ 4 day- and summer-sanatoria	206
„ 4 private sanatoria	331
	8,608

This is equivalent to 104 beds for every 100 deaths from tuberculosis.

The State grants up to 2,000 kroner per bed for new buildings; and gives a daily grant for maintenance of each patient in a recognised institution of 1.75 to 1.25 kroner.

At institutions provided by county councils and municipalities patients usually pay 1 krone a day, but are admitted free if without means.[1]

In Stockholm, at the municipal dispensaries, 7,392 patients were examined in 1928, of whom 2,410 were new patients, and 8,037 domiciliary visits were made. Help was given to tuberculous patients at a cost of over 152,000 kroner. At these tuberculosis dispensaries patients are only received who are sent by a physician. They thus differ essentially from a polyclinic. Dr. Kjellin, the head of one of these dispensaries, stated that special work was being done in the

---

[1] *The Official Hospital Organisation in Sweden*, No. 59, Stockholm, 1929.

examination of each member of affected families, and that work on a considerable scale was being done in the segregation of infants and young children from infected patients. Where possible this was done for three years—one at home, and two years in the country.

New-born children of tuberculous mothers were also separated from the parents, who are said to permit this in 95 per cent. of the cases.

PATHOLOGICAL WORK

To a certain extent pathological work is undertaken throughout Sweden for medical practitioners without their paying therefor. In Stockholm, in the municipal bacteriological laboratory, 8,284 specimens of material from suspected diphtheria were examined in 1928, in addition to 887 specimens for tuberculosis and 330 Wassermann tests.

ANTI-ALCOHOLIC WORK

Sweden has been the home of interesting pioneer efforts to reduce alcoholism. For much information on this subject I am indebted to Rev. David Ostlund, who is the leading advocate in Sweden of more stringent measures than those already taken.

The evil is one of great magnitude in all Scandinavian countries, and especially in Sweden, though much less so than a hundred years ago, when there was very general drunkenness. At that time spirits were distilled in nearly every farm in the country. In 1829 the consumption of brandy was 46 litres *per cap.*, as shown by the taxation on the known manufacture of spirits. Then started the Swedish temperance movement under the famous Dean Wieselgram, which led in 1855 to the Swedish Diet prohibiting home distillation, and placing the manufacture of spirits in the hands of a few State bodies. In 1860–65 the consumption of spirits had fallen to 11 litres *per cap.*

In the last-named year the Göteborg system was established in that city, which removed the element of private profit. The misdemeanours due to drink greatly declined under this system. But its effect was limited in the main to the sale of potato spirit, while cognac and whisky soon found a Swedish market, and all wines were allowed. There was the further objection that the municipality benefited in public works from the profits of the trade in spirits, which fact did not increase municipal enthusiasm for a restricted sale.

In 1909 occurred a General Strike in Sweden, during which total prohibition was enforced by the Government for six weeks; and this was followed by a plebiscite of the people, organised by temperance societies, on prohibition. There were 1,900,000 votes for and 17,000 against national prohibition. Of the total population aged eighteen and over 99 per cent. at that time favoured prohibition.

Dr. Bratt at this time began to write in favour of an alternative system of rationing the individual supply of alcohol by means of a "Motbook", and eventually the "Bratt system" was adopted. Each orderly person is given this passport, authorising him or her to purchase 4 litres of spirit each month ($4\frac{1}{2}$ litres = 1 gallon). This system has worked on the whole smoothly. It appears to be successful in preventing the socialising of drinking, which is a chief cause of excess. It does not, however, reduce the average consumption in the community by those who never get drunk, but may nevertheless be intemperate.

In 1922 Sweden consumed 27,700,000 litres of brandy, while in 1929, with almost no increase of population in the interval, she consumed 32,080,000 litres.

Under the Bratt system the number of consumers is steadily increasing, and the system has had a curious psychological effect. The possession of a passport or Motbook is being regarded almost as a testimonial of trustworthy character, and is valued accordingly.

To sum up, if the prevention of drunkenness were the sole object, the Bratt system presents good features, but it is well-known that the greater part of the mischief done by alcohol is unassociated with actual intoxication.

At present there is a widespread movement in Sweden to secure a system of local option for each district to control the local sale of drink, and to secure greatly increased taxation of spirits, to an extent which will decrease its consumption.

CHAPTER IV

NORWAY[1]

PRELIMINARY SUMMARY

The medical organisation of Norway presents features of much interest.

The provision in each district of a district medical officer and an official midwife ensures medical and obstetric care to a large proportion of the total population; and this provision continues, as in the past, to be a guarantee against medical neglect.

The arrangements for the compulsory sickness insurance of wage-earners and for their medical care have an instructive bearing on the general problem of medical attendance.

Hospital treatment is provided on a large scale, and, as in other Scandinavian countries, charges are made according to means. All hospital provision is made by official authorities.

The long-continued practice in Norway of requiring all private medical practitioners and all hospitals to transmit periodical returns of cases treated by them is deserving of general adoption.

The low rate of mortality from causes associated with pregnancy and childbirth is noteworthy, an experience for which the almost universal employment of trained midwives must be held largely responsible.

Norway is a sparsely-populated country, and its people are relatively poor. Distances are great, and transport very difficult. It is as far from Oslo to the North Cape as from Oslo to Rome, and takes longer to reach the most northerly point of Norway than to cross the Atlantic.

These facts help to show that its admirable system for ensuring medical provision for its people could only be possible by means of well-organised communal co-operation.

Norway consists largely of barren and mountainous country. Its area is 124,964 square miles, of which about 29,000 are forest. Of its total area only 3·2 per cent. is under

[1] Date of investigation, July 1930.

cultivation, while 24·2 per cent. is forest, and the rest unproductive. Its forests constitute one of its chief natural sources of wealth, next to these coming its fisheries. Its enormous water-power has aided in the development of other industries.

The Norwegian krone (100 öre) is equal to about 13½ English pence, or 27 American cents.

GOVERNMENT

The union of Norway and Sweden was dissolved in 1905. The Storting is the representative governing body; but the King has the power to veto Acts passed by this body, until these have been confirmed at two general elections. Every man and woman aged twenty-three and over has a vote in the election of the 150 members of the Storting. Proportional representation is adopted, the country for this purpose being divided into districts, each of which elects three to eight representatives.

The Storting, when elected, divides itself into two houses, the Lagting and the Odelsting, the former comprising one-fourth and the latter three-fourths of the elected members. If the two houses disagree on a proposal a joint meeting of both is held, and a two-thirds majority of the two houses thus sitting decides. The members are paid a salary.

The Government executive is a cabinet or council of State, consisting of the Prime Minister and seven other ministers. Ministers attend the Storting but cannot vote. The Minister for Social Affairs has charge of medical and public health matters.

Local Government.—Norway is divided into 20 districts, of which Oslo and Bergen form two. These districts comprise 43 towns, 24 ports, and 674 rural communes (*herreder*).

Each *herred* has 12 to 48 elected representatives, who appoint a council consisting of a fourth of their number. The towns and ports form 65 additional communes.

The communes have a high degree of autonomy, except

in the appointment of their health officers. Each commune
has a health council, presided over by the district medical
officer, who is appointed by royal decree.

The estimated population of Norway in 1928 was
2,787,827, of which 785,404 were in towns. Oslo's population in 1920 was 258,483.

THE MEDICAL PROFESSION

At the end of 1927 Norway had 1,674 doctors, 892 dentists, and 1,070 students of medicine. The training of doctors
occupies seven years, and all students are examined in
hygiene and public health.

Out of the total number of doctors some 400 are engaged
in public health work, most of them as part-time officers.

Each town with a population exceeding 15,000 has a
stadsfysikus. In smaller towns and rural districts the public
medical officer is called a *stadslege*.

This medical officer is the key to the entire medical work
in each commune. He cannot be removed from office and
is pensionable. He supervises the medical practitioners,
pharmacists, dentists, midwives, and assistant vaccinators
of the district.

He receives the weekly notifications of certain diseases
required from medical practitioners, and transmits these,
and in addition makes an annual general report on general
health conditions, to the Health Officer of the county or
prefecture in which his commune is situate. The medical
officer of the prefecture is usually a full-time officer, and he
is required to report to the Central Ministry. Occasionally
he also acts as district medical officer. All the local medical
officers in Norway are under the control of the Central
Ministry, of which Dr. Wefring is the chief medical officer.
Their appointment is made by the Central Ministry. Usually
three names are submitted by the council of the county or
prefecture, one of the three being chosen by the Ministry.
To Dr. Wefring I am indebted for the information on this
and allied subjects, though I am alone responsible for any
expression of opinions.

Most of the district medical officers are engaged also in private medical practice, and, in addition to their public health and other supervisory work, in rural districts they are responsible also for the medical care of poor persons. This treatment is required from the medical officers at their dispensaries and within three kilometres from the medical officer's home without remuneration apart from their official salary. For distances exceeding three kilometres they receive 6 kroner, which is paid by the local authority, for visits not exceeding one in twenty-four hours. Further travelling allowances are fixed according to an official tariff, and are paid by the State. In the smaller towns the State pays one-third and the town two-thirds of the urban medical officer's fixed salary. No additional payment is received usually for treating indigent patients, but the municipality may give additional remuneration for this. In larger towns with a population exceeding 15,000 the *stadsfysikus* has not the duty of treating the poor, and special medical officers are appointed for this work by the municipality. In Oslo there are no special medical officers for the treatment of the sick poor; these have a free choice of doctors, who are paid according to service rendered.

In each area there is an officer who decides on the suitability of recipients for medical aid. This intermediation is dispensed with in medical emergencies.

Of the total population of Norway it is estimated that some 400,000, or about 14 per cent., are medically attended gratuitously by the district medical officer. In the north it may be more than this, in the south less. It appears likely that half of the total medical attendance of the community, including hospitals and sickness insurance, is at least partially at the expense of communal funds.

The district medical officer's work is supplemented by the provision of general hospital treatment.

HOSPITALS

In 1927 there were 175 general hospitals having 10,742 available beds. In addition, there were 4,376 beds for tuberculosis, 305 for lying-in hospitals, 138 for leprosy, 120 for alcoholics, and 5,368 for the insane. There were 489 additional beds for epileptics and feeble-minded. Leprosy is now nearly extinct. Lepers without children are allowed to remain at home if they live under favourable conditions.

The larger hospitals have been provided by the county councils (prefectures). There is one State general hospital, the Rikshospital in Oslo, which acts as the University clinic for medical students. At this hospital the heads of each department are University professors in the Faculty of Medicine. The State has also provided a special clinic for cripples in Oslo. At the State hospital a very small fee is charged to patients, the deficit being borne by the State. At municipal and county hospitals somewhat larger fees are charged, the deficit being borne by public funds.

In rural districts there may be no hospital, except for infectious diseases; but hospital accommodation is always available in a neighbouring community.

Insurance societies do not pay more for insured patients admitted to hospital than others are charged. A higher charge is usually made for patients from other districts than that in which the county or district hospital is situate. The rate of payment ranges from 3 kroner up to 9 or 10 kroner per diem for ordinary treatment. In most hospitals it is 5 or 6 kroner a day, including medicine, dressings, and medical attendance. In Oslo the charge per diem for hospital treatment for insured and non-insured alike is 3 kroner. The same payment is made by well-to-do; but they may pay more for a special room. Some doctors expressed to me the opinion that there is over-resort to hospitals.

Norway has practically no voluntary hospitals supported out of charitable funds.

The medical staff of hospitals receive salaries from the municipality, county council, or State, as the case may be. The hospital doctor also receives a fee for each surgical operation. Physicians, as a rule, receive no extra payment beyond their salaries, but they can have private practice. An instance was given of a hospital surgeon in a suburb of Oslo who receives a salary of 30,000 kroner. He is also allowed private practice, but has little time for this.

There are no polyclinics at the hospitals in Oslo comparable to those in Stockholm, to which any person can come for a payment of 2 kroner a visit; and thus one great source of medical friction is avoided.

MIDWIVES

Every district in Norway is provided with an official midwife as well as with an official medical attendant for the poor. For midwifery the country is divided into 1,000 districts, some of its 739 communes or districts having more than one official midwife. In 1925 there were 1,534 midwives, of whom 1,000 were official. These are required to give their services gratuitously to the poor, although they may also have private patients.

Each midwife since 1888 has been required to graduate from a midwifery school at Oslo or at Bergen. The course of training only lasts a year. Midwives are not allowed to perform operations. Some of them, but not all, are also fully trained nurses. Great cleanliness is practised; and their services are called for not only gratuitously for the poor, but by all classes of the community. In 1927 the proportion of the total 50,999 births in Norway attended by midwives was 93·3 per cent.

There is an increasing tendency to be confined in the midwifery section of a general hospital or in a special lying-in hospital. In Oslo over half the total births occur in hospitals.

Doctors express no objection to the almost complete monopoly of normal midwifery by midwives. It has never been otherwise.

The salary of a midwife varies according to the prospect of additional private practice. Two-fifths of the salary is paid by the State, two-fifths by the county, and one-fifth by the commune. In towns the midwives' salaries are paid out of municipal funds. Each midwife is pensionable.

If a woman who has not been granted public assistance

is attended by the official midwife, the latter can demand a fee, but its amount is fixed by the prefect of the county.

Midwives may be suspended from practice either by the district or county medical officer.

VACCINATION

This forms an additional source of income for certain midwives, who have been specially instructed in this work, in accordance with a very old practice. In rural areas these selected midwives do most of the vaccination against smallpox. In remote districts this is carried out in the schools once a year, or biennially, mothers bringing their children for this purpose. Nominally no compulsion is exercised; but as a child cannot be confirmed in church or be received into the higher school, and, further, cannot afterwards be married by the parish minister, unless vaccinated, formal compulsion is unneeded.

Midwives are supplied with vaccine lymph, and they are paid half a krone for each certificate of vaccination. No further fee is paid. The midwife who undertakes vaccination has to be specially appointed by the prefect of the county.

Here, again, no objection is raised by the doctors; and this is a useful indication of the extent to which medical services are expected to be provided by public authorities.

Private doctors also vaccinate, where payment can be obtained. In Oslo facilities for public vaccination are provided twice a week. There is much vaccination of sailors to avoid quarantine restrictions.

SICKNESS INSURANCE MEDICAL WORK

Since 1911, the year when the English system was introduced, there has been compulsory sickness insurance in Norway for wage-earners and for non-manual workers earning less than 6,000 kroner a year (i.e. about £270, or $1,350), and these may continue to be insured voluntarily when their earnings rise above this level. The limiting income has now been lowered to 5,200 kroner.

About 23 per cent. of the total population is insured. This figure does not include the wives and children of the insured. Including them the proportion is increased to between 50 and 60 per cent.

Sickness benefit begins after three days' incapacity for work, and amounts to 60 per cent. of the average daily earnings of the class to which the person insured belongs. In 1924,[1] on an average, each insured person had 9·84 days of sickness in the year, including the first three days of sickness.

The sick person is entitled to medical treatment, and to supply of certain appliances, as spectacles or trusses. Since 1929 appliances, including spectacles and trusses, are not supplied under the benefit; and dental treatment does not include artificial teeth or fillings, but only extraction of teeth. The insurance doctor must give medical treatment to the wife and family of the insured, including dependents up to the age of fifteen. Drugs are not an insurable benefit. In 1924[2] the total expenditure per member was distributed in the following proportions :—

14·7 per cent. for hospital treatment,
26·6 per cent. for medical fees,
2·1 per cent. for dental fees,
3·5 per cent. for medical appliances, baths, etc.,
3·8 per cent. for travelling expenses of doctors and patients,
5·0 per cent, for maternity benefit,
8·5 per cent. for administration.

This leaves 35·8 per cent of the total expenditure for monetary benefits. The administrative cost is stated to be a less proportion of the total funds than in England.

Insured women receive a lying-in benefit, which includes payment for free attendance by a midwife, in accordance with a specified scale, and a money maternity benefit for six weeks after confinement. Sometimes these benefits are given to the uninsured wives of insured men. Hospital treatment may be substituted for a midwife.

[1] *Compulsory Sickness Insurance* (League of Nations publication, 1927). [2] Ibid.

Payment of Insurance Doctors.—For much information under this heading I am indebted to Dr. Jorgen Berner, the able secretary of the Norwegian Medical Association. Dr. Berner was formerly a district medical officer, and was able to throw much light on the absence of friction between these district officers and private doctors. The sparse population goes far to explain this good working. The district medical officer may be the only doctor in his district. The difference between England and Norway may be illustrated by insurance data quoted by Dr. Berner.

In England there are 65 insured persons for every square kilometre.

In Denmark there are 35 insured persons for every square kilometre.

In Norway there is 1 insured person for every square kilometre.

The insured person in Norway has a free choice of doctor, and the doctor can accept or decline a patient. The Medical Association lays stress on payment for each service rendered by the doctor, and on the doctor being allowed to charge for this service an amount which he thinks appropriate. If this amount exceeds the amount allowed by the insurance society, the patient pays the doctor the difference. Insurance societies pay 3.50 kroner for each consultation, and 5 kroner for a medical visit in Oslo, but the doctor is usually paid 5 and 7 kroner for these by the insured. In Bergen doctors have agreed to a payment of 4 kroner, and in other districts 3.50 kroner is paid for the first consultation. The agreed tariff after the first consultation is 2 kroner for the second, and 1.50 kroner for subsequent consultations, with an additional allowance for travelling. Special fees are fixed for special work. The Norwegian method of payment is less remunerative in rural districts, owing to sparsity of population and the long distances to be travelled. In the towns it works well, but the insured are dissatisfied because of the difference between the doctor's fee and what is refunded by the society.

Travelling expenses are allowed in addition to the fixed payment per visit:—

For a distance of	1 kilometre	..	5 kroner.
,,	3	,,	6 ,,
,,	5	,,	7 ,,
,,	7	,,	8 ,,
,,	10	,,	9 ,,

The doctor is paid by the insured person, who then obtains vouchers from the doctor, in return for which he receives the multiple of 5 kroner which he owes the doctor. In this process the doctor may sometimes fail to be paid.

As elsewhere, doctors are apt to grumble at the medical certificates required from them, for which no separate payment is made. In rural districts, again, there are occasional complaints because the patient will not pay more than the official scale of charge. The above system was only adopted three years ago; prior to that there was the same system as in Denmark.

The method of payment outlined above is liked by the doctors. A different opinion is held by insurance societies, especially in towns. According to them, in rural districts the method does not appear to work unsatisfactorily. In towns it is not so satisfactory.

In discussing the method of paying doctors with representatives of insurance and medicine respectively, I was impressed by the identity of English and Norwegian insurance problems. According to the capitation basis holding good in England, the tendency is for each patient to receive less attention, and according to the Norwegian system to receive more attention, than is required in his medical interest. The English system presents the great advantage that the conscientious doctor can give all the attention he thinks his patient needs, without suspicion of unworthy motives. It has the disadvantage that the "slacker" may neglect his patient by hasty or imperfect work, or by scanty attendance, without adequate control. In Norway the patient has to pay for drugs, and I was assured that if drugs were to be supplied to insured patients by the insurance societies, associated doctors would at once require a fee 25 per cent. higher than at present. This responsible statement, I think, is very significant. The liability of the patient to pay for drugs gives him a motive for discouraging that over-medication and unnecessary prescribing, without which in England patients often are dissatisfied; and it gives the intelligent doctor an opportunity of teaching each patient the greater value of regimen and hygiene than of drugs. Unless this counsel is given, the insured person's obligation to pay for drugs may lead to his not seeking medical advice when it is desirable. But notwithstanding this regulation as to drugs, overuse of medical aid is complained of by some insurance societies.

In 1928, the last year for which statistics are available, the cost of medical treatment in Norway was 14.2 kroner (i.e. about 16s., or less than $4), compared with 9s. in England. In this sum in Norway is included medical treatment not only to the insured, but also to his family, and there are provided all kinds of special services, including skilled attendance in childbirth.

Which system is best for the patient? In Norway the patient may restrict undue activity of his doctor, and thus save himself expense for medicines. The patient thus becomes a partial check on the exceptional mercenary doctor. In England the only check against the neglect which occasionally occurs—whether in actual failure to respond to calls or in incomplete care in diagnosis—is the patient's desire to change his doctor if neglected. The patient's prejudice or ignorance leaves this a very fortuitous protection. He is perhaps more likely to change from a competent and conscientious doctor than from a plausible practitioner, too facile in giving and continuing certificates of incapacity for work. The medical profession in Norway are definitely of opinion that for the maintenance of a high standard of medical work the Norwegian system of payment is superior to that of Denmark and England. At the same time they recognise that complete treatment, as given in

Norway, must be expensive, and that the demands of patients steadily increase.

It is possible that medical men in Norway would not be unwilling to go back to the capitation system, if the tariff were made high enough, but this is not really favoured by most doctors. In one small town it had been introduced by way of trial. In this town medical payment is fixed at 15 kroner per head, for married and unmarried alike.

Hospital treatment is usually paid for by insurance societies at its full cost.

Insurance Societies.—As in England, sickness insurance grew up gradually under private management. I am indebted to Dr. Ing Per Larssen, Director of the Central Office for Social Insurance, for much information which follows. Ninety-two per cent. of the insured in insurance societies in Norway are incorporated in this central society. Altogether there are 754 kassen or insurance societies, besides thirty-eight private societies under Government inspection. Only one kasse is allowed in each district, unless specially sanctioned; and this kasse deals not only with sickness insurance, but also with invalidity insurance and old age pensions. Thus there is no competition between different societies, and uniformity of administration is facilitated.

The expense of sickness insurance is borne to the extent of six-tenths by the insured person; the employer pays one-tenth, the commune one-tenth, and the State two-tenths. (In Denmark the State pays nothing, except indirectly in partial maintenance of hospitals.) It is noteworthy that the proportion insured is higher in Denmark with voluntary than in Norway with compulsory insurance.

The Central Office for Sickness Insurance also has charge of invalidity and accident insurance. Its staff includes five physicians, one concerned with sickness and four with accident work. The employer pays the entire premium for accident insurance. Since the Great War claims for accident insurance have become excessive. This has not resulted largely from malingering, though lack of employment tends to increase claims and to prolong incapacity. Patients are sent to specialists in their own area, and to hospitals for observation.

Both in accident insurance and in sickness insurance claims increase when economic conditions are unfavourable. The great problem in insurance in Norway, as elsewhere, is to convince the insured that apart from the actual exigencies for which insurance has been effected, it is not really advantageous to the insured, and is not "playing the game", to make unnecessary claims, or to retain benefits for a larger period than is necessary.

MATERNITY AND CHILD WELFARE

The Norwegian birth-rate in 1927 was 17·8 per 1,000, as compared with 19·5 in 1925, still-births (from the twenty-eighth week of pregnancy) forming 2·4 per cent. of total births. Illegitimate births form about 7 per cent. of the total live-births.

In Oslo in 1927 the birth-rate was only 9·0; in Bergen it was 14·9.

Infant mortality in 1927 for the whole of Norway was 51·1 per 1,000 live-births, as compared with 63·1 in 1918. It has remained at about its present level during the last four years.

PUERPERAL MORTALITY

The statistics of mortality in child-bearing are important, even if a measure of doubt be entertained as to their complete accuracy, a doubt which emerges in the corresponding statistics of other countries. As the International Classification of Causes of Death is used in Scandinavian countries, doubt can only arise on the assumption of varying exactitude of doctors when signing death certificates in revealing the association of death with parturition or abortion, and subsequent variation in the classification of death returns. It may be added here that as the birth-rate is somewhat low, and especially so in Oslo, this implies a high proportion of primiparæ, among whom complications of parturition are more frequent than in multiparæ. As this is a phenomenon common to nearly all Western European countries, it is not likely to vitiate greatly approximate comparisons of puerperal mortality, though it has a disturbing influence on comparisons with the past. It may also affect the comparisons between Oslo and Norway as a whole given below.

In the five years 1923–27 total puerperal mortality in Norway varied between 3·2 and 2·4 per 1,000 births, the last figure relating to 1927. In country districts in the same period the rate varied between 2·7 and 2·3, and in towns between 4·3 and 2·9. Thus there was always some excess in towns as compared with other parts of Norway. In the following table a similar comparison, with the addition of the figures for Oslo, is made for 1927. The small numbers upon which the higher rates for Oslo are based will be noted, as well as the remark in the last paragraph.

PUERPERAL MORTALITY, 1927.

	Births	Number of Deaths from		Death-rate per 1,000 Births	
		Puerperal Sepsis	Other Causes of Puerperal Mortality	Puerperal Sepsis	Other Causes of Puerperal Mortality
Norway ..	50,260	51	72	1·01	1·43
Towns ..	10,633	14	19	1·32	1·78
Oslo	2,312	5	9	2·16	1·73
Rural districts	39,627	37	53	0·99	1·33

There can be no hesitation in attributing the low general rate of puerperal mortality in Norway to the efficient midwifery service of the country, supported as it is by adequate medical help when needed, including hospital provision in a large proportion of cases. The experience of towns is less favourable than that of the rest of Norway, and that of Oslo is the least favourable. In Oslo in 1927 the crude birth-rate was only half that for the whole of Norway, which means a larger proportion of first-births, in which the risks of parturition are greater than—perhaps double —the risks at next succeeding births. This will explain some of the difference. In view of the more abundant institutional provision of Oslo, some of this statistical handicap should be balanced. It will be noted, furthermore, that the excess in deaths from sepsis is great in towns, and especially in Oslo.

Some light is thrown on the problem by the fact that, comparing (a) all districts outside towns with (b) the aggregate experience of Norwegian towns, in 1927 the recorded deaths give the following contrast:—

	In (a)	In (b)
The deaths from puerperal sepsis at term..	33	6
The deaths from puerperal sepsis in abortions	4	8
The deaths from all other causes of puerperal mortality	53	19

It is evident that abortion associated with sepsis is more frequent in towns than in rural districts, and it is likely that this may have borne a larger share than the figures reveal in raising the urban puerperal mortality. If this can be verified by more detailed and exact returns, it is evident that comparisons of mortality from puerperal sepsis will need to be considered in relation to the amount of abortion in each community. It may occur, for instance, that even a relatively low puerperal mortality associated with a specially efficient—including a more completely aseptic —midwifery service fails to reveal the full extent of the superiority of its service on account of widespread practice of intentional abortion.

It is probable that this is the case both in Copenhagen and Stockholm, and to some extent in Oslo.

Child Welfare Work

There is no general system of home visitation of infants, except on the occurrence of an epidemic disease. Special care is taken of illegitimate children, and paternity is investigated, with a view to the father supporting the child.

School Medical Work

Compulsory school attendance begins at the age of seven, and throughout each school year a large proportion of scholars get a free meal.

In Oslo there has been a special school medical department since December 1918. Its chief medical officer, Dr. Carl Schotz, is a full-time officer, acting jointly under the School Board and the Board of Health. Under him are thirty-one school doctors, one being attached to every one of the twenty public schools and the six higher schools in the city. In addition, the school staff includes a medical specialist for throat, one for eye cases, and one for the feeble-minded. Each of the school doctors is engaged also in private practice, but is expected to devote an hour a week to each school. No treatment is undertaken for children found to need it. Patients are referred to a private doctor, and each case is re-inspected by the school doctor and nurse. If the patient's parents cannot afford treatment, this is given at the expense of the municipality.

No objection is made by private doctors to the limited medical supervision undertaken in the schools.

On leaving school each pupil is invited to a voluntary examination with a view to suitable choice of occupation, and 67 per cent. of the boys and 62 per cent. of the girls on leaving the elementary schools in 1929 presented themselves for this examination, a smaller proportion in the secondary and higher schools. All children in whose families there is tuberculosis are examined by the school doctor. There are summer colonies at which places are found for 2,000, or about 8·5 per cent., of the elementary school children each year. Each scholar is measured and weighed before and after this vacation.

TUBERCULOSIS

The large amount of institutional provision has already been indicated. Insurance societies defray the cost of treatment of a large number of patients, who but for this provision would depend on the funds for public assistance.

Two national voluntary associations engage in anti-tuberculosis work, including the establishment of tuberculosis dispensaries, the provision of visiting nurses in the communes, etc. Dispensaries are few in number.

The Norwegian death-rate from tuberculosis is high, 1·33 per 1,000 in 1927. It is significant that the female is higher than the male death-rate from this disease, a position which held good for England and some other countries in years before active preventive work was general.

In 1927 the deaths from all forms of tuberculosis in Norway numbered 4,460, and in the same year 7,091 cases were notified in accordance with the obligation imposed by the law.

The death-rate from pulmonary tuberculosis in 1927 was 1·40 per 1,000 in Oslo; the lowest death-rate was 0·77 in Opland, the highest, 2·33, in Finnmark.

The central Government contributes to some tuberculosis activities, including the maintenance of sanatorium beds. The funds for this purpose are derived largely from a national lottery. In Oslo fifteen nurses are employed by the municipality for home visitation to tuberculous patients.

There is evidently much scope for further active anti-tuberculosis work in Norway.

VENEREAL DISEASES

There is no special organisation for the treatment of venereal patients. Outside the larger towns there are no special facilities for the treatment of these diseases. There is much venereal disease in seaports, and gratuitous treatment is given in Bergen and Oslo. Most patients go to private doctors or to the district medical officers.

Returns are made of the number of cases of venereal diseases treated in hospitals, and from these tables given in

Sundhetstilstanden og Medisinalforholdene, 1927, the following figures have been extracted:—

506 cases of syphilis,
557 cases of gonorrhœa.

These figures give the total new cases treated in 20 hospitals. Of the above total, 249 cases of syphilis and 309 cases of gonorrhœa were treated in Oslo, and 42 cases of syphilis and 31 cases of gonorrhœa in Bergen.

With these figures may be compared the cases of these two diseases notified in the twenty prefectures in Norway, in accordance with the general duty imposed on doctors.

	Number of Cases notified during 1927	
	Syphilis	Gonorrhœa
Rural districts ..	185	1,114
Towns	1,269	5,870

There is no provision for the gratuitous supply of arsenobenzol preparations, except in so far as district medical officers use it in their practice among the poor, and its further use in hospitals.

VITAL STATISTICS

Although Norway had records of births and deaths at an earlier date than most European countries, its records are not so complete, nor did they begin so early as those of Sweden. As in Sweden, the clergy kept lists of births, deaths, and marriages, and from 1800 the registration of still-births was added. From the year 1814, when Norway separated from Denmark, the collation of the Norwegian statistics came under the central department of finance; and in 1837, in the year in which national vital statistics began, a Norwegian statistical bureau was established.

In 1896, in a paper entitled "A National System of

Notification and Registration of Sickness"(*Journ. Roy. Statist. Soc.*, vol. lix. Part 1), I described the system of notification of cases of sickness in vogue in Scandinavian countries. This, then as now, presented features worthy of imitation by other countries. I do not propose to enter into details here, but the following points are noteworthy. There is immediate notification of certain diseases, while weekly or monthly returns are required from each doctor of new cases which have come under his care. It is evident that in obtaining these returns the fact that in every parish a large share of medical practice is conducted by the official district medical officer makes the task exceptionally easy. As in other countries (except in Great Britain), no payment is made to the doctor for these returns. Returns of hospital cases are made as well as of cases in private practice.

The list of diseases returned weekly or monthly does not give names and addresses, while in the immediate notification of the chief infectious diseases these and other particulars are required. The periodical statistical returns include, among other diseases, venereal diseases, pleurisy and other respiratory diseases, influenza, acute gastroenteritis, and rheumatic fever.

CHAPTER V

GERMANY[1]

PRELIMINARY SUMMARY

Germany is a federation of States with varying medical conditions, but all subject to the federal Sickness Insurance Act.

Special doctors for the poor have been replaced partially by insurance doctors. Hospitals are chiefly national or municipal institutions, supported by taxation, assisted by payment according to means and from insurance funds. Social welfare organisations are many, and their functioning such as to call for co-ordination and partial fusion. Much social welfare work is carried on by insurance organisations parallel with that of public health authorities. Similar inco-ordination, partial or entire, exists in tuberculosis and anti-venereal work.

Medical attendance for a majority of the total population is under the National Sickness Insurance scheme. Most insurance societies provide medical treatment for the dependents of the insured. The treatment includes the services of specialists and often hospital treatment. The contracts of doctors with insurance societies are on varying bases. There is a vast amount of medical dissatisfaction as to the conditions of insurance work.

For special conditions in Hamburg, see page 180.

GENERAL CONDITIONS

The circumstances of private and public medical practice throughout Germany are as complex as its systems of central and local government; and it is necessary to envisage the latter if we are to understand the problems of medicine. Medicine, indeed, is one of the chief problems of government, primarily and chiefly owing to Germany's systems of sickness, invalidity, and accident insurance, but also very largely as a consequence of the great extent to which public

Date of investigation, June 1929.

health authorities have undertaken work for the protection of maternity and child welfare and for the treatment and prevention of sickness in the poor, and, so far as infectious diseases are concerned, in the entire population.

The republic of Germany consists of eighteen federal States having in 1925 a population of about 63½ millions, of whom 61 per cent. belonged to Prussia, 11·8 per cent. to Bavaria, 4·1 per cent. to Württemberg, 3·7 per cent. to Baden, 8·0 per cent. to Saxony, 1·9 per cent. to Hamburg, and the rest to smaller States of the republic.

A Council of the States (Reichsrat) represents the component States, and the consent of the Reichsrat is required for the introduction of proposed legislation into the Reichstag, or National Assembly, which is elected on the basis of proportional representation by adult German suffrage (men and women). The Reichstag is elected for four years, and it can pass Bills by a majority of two-thirds over the head of the Reichsrat.

The largest city in Germany is Berlin, which in 1925 had a population of 4,024,165; Hamburg, the next largest city at the same date, having a population of 1,079,126.

In accordance with Article 7 of the German Constitution of August 11, 1919, the Government of the Reich, the entity formed by the eighteen constituent States, has legislative authority throughout Germany, *inter alia*, in regard to matters affecting the population and its health, and especially the care of mothers, nurslings, children, and the young.

Questions of health are dealt with mainly by the

> Reich Ministry of the Interior, and
> The Reich Ministry of Labour.

Health matters are administered chiefly in two departments of the Ministry of the Interior. Department II is concerned with

> Public health,
> Sanitary, police and hygiene,
> Questions of medical staff,
> Medical examinations and investigations,

Infant mortality,
Tuberculosis,
Alcoholic excess,
Training of doctors, pharmacists, etc.

Department III of the Ministry of the Interior deals with

Popular education,
Child welfare,
Physical training.

The Reich Ministry of Labour is concerned with

Matters affecting the care of workers,
Welfare institutions,
Other questions of social policy, e.g.
    Insurance of workers,
    Care of unemployed,
    Maintenance of disabled soldiers and widows and orphans,
    Industrial hygiene.

The *Reich Health Office* guides the Minister in matters of public health. This office is divided into four chief sections:

Medical,
Chemical,
Bacteriological, and
Veterinary.

This office has as its auxiliary the *Reich Health Council*, an advisory body of some seventy-five members, chosen by the Reichsrat for five years from various expert services and scientific fields; and this Council is divided into eleven committees, for the consideration of various problems.[1]

Prussia, the largest German State, may be taken as an example of State health organisation. The organisation of other German States is on somewhat similar lines.

The formation of the republic in 1919 left to each State the power to regulate its own systems of local government, subject to federal law. In each State education is under direct State control. In each State there are two distinct but parallel forms of local government, viz. State functions

[1] For further particulars, Dr. Gottfried's contribution on the *Public Health Services in Germany* (League of Nations publication) may be consulted.

carried out by officers and bodies directly responsible to the *State Health Council* (corresponding to the Reich Health Council), and the self-government of communes and other areas by directly elected local authorities. The representatives on these are elected by universal adult suffrage, as for the Reichstag. In Prussia the health officers are under the Ministry of Public Welfare, instead of a State Health Council; the latter is purely advisory.

Three orders of local authorities exist.

The *province*, includes both the town and rural circles within it.

Next comes the *circle* (Kreis), with, in addition, independent (Kreisfrei) towns above a certain population.

The unit of local self-government is the *commune* (Gemeinde), which may be rural (Landgemeinde) or urban (Stadt). In 1925 the number of communes in Germany was 63,580.

Each of these usually is controlled by a directly representative body and has an executive organ. In rural communes the head man (Vorsteher), and in towns the burgomaster or *Magistrat* (a Board appointed by the Town Council), form the executive. The executive, whether personal or a committee, whether salaried or not, is usually professional, and is largely independent of the elective body. This is the outstanding distinction from methods of English local government, where local patriotism has hitherto provided local citizens who have been willing to undertake time-consuming services on the local authority, as chairman, mayor, or in other capacities.

The burgomaster commonly holds office for twelve years, and may be re-elected for life. He is salaried, and is the real agent of local administration.

Each circle or commune has a Landrat, who is chairman of the local elected council, and is chosen by them. The Landrat, or in Kreisfrei towns the burgomaster, is a State officer, largely independent of the district or town council.

In each Landrat's office in towns there is a *Welfare Office*, for which there is no statutory sanction. Youth Offices (Jugendämter) are required to be established by the federal law of July 1922 in all districts; and Welfare Offices embracing the welfare of the young with other activities are general. They include economic, educational, and health divisions, the second of these undertaking care of the young. To it have gradually become attached Fürsorgerinnen, i.e. female officers charged with this care. These are usually inadequate in number. Voluntary workers supplement their efforts. Commonly there is a separate Welfare Director under the Landrat, who has charge of destitution, while a special syndicate deals with education, and the district or communal medical officer deals with health problems.

In towns the communal medical officer is often called the Stadt Medizinalrat; he directs the activities of the physicians engaged in care of infants, tuberculosis work, school work, and all needing medical certification.

State circle medical officers are required to pass a State examination; while communal medical officers need only take a three months' course of supplementary training at one of the three Social Hygiene Academies in Berlin—Charlottenburg, Breslau, Düsseldorf.

Commissioners are appointed to advise the Landrat or burgomaster on various health and other problems.

Statistics can only be given for Prussia. In 1925 this State had 449 Kreis medical officers, of whom 274 received full-time and 175 only part-time salaries; but now they are all full-time officers. They comprise 432 medical officers and 34 medical assessors. The Kreis medical officer may be required to do other work of an official character. As a rule these medical officers are required to pass a State examination as a condition of appointment.

All "police" matters, interpreted in a wide sense, are reserved by the State, the local executive or burgomaster being responsible for their actual exercise.

The extent to which other—including public health—functions are delegated to local authorities varies greatly. In the large towns this may be almost complete, and many of these towns have built up admirable independent public health and medical services.

All local authorities, however, are subject to State control, to ensure that action is in all respects in accordance with the law, and in certain matters there is Imperial (Reich) control. State and local authorities cannot levy an income tax, but States and, through them, the communes receive a portion of the produce of imperial taxation. The States and communes can impose land, house and industrial taxes.

PRUSSIA

The central health authority in Prussia is the *Ministry of Public Welfare*, which has three departments:—

1. Public health, including police and sanitary regulations, with a doctor at its head;
2. Housing and land settlement;
3. Care of the young and general welfare work.

Attached to these are various institutes (including the Robert Koch Institute for Infectious Diseases) and laboratories.

Prussia is now divided into 14 *provinces*, each of these being subdivided into *Government districts*, and these again into *circles*.

In 1921 there were 430 circles in Prussia, and 106 municipalities independent of the circle authorities.

As in the rest of Germany, there is the dual organisation of elected local representatives and of a local executive representing the State. The Government President of each district covering a number of circles (Regierungs-Präsident) is appointed by the central Government. He presides over the Government Board (Regierung), consisting of professional officials.

In the province a similar arrangement exists, the Chief President (Ober-präsident) having even more power than a French Prefect.

Of the representative local bodies, the most important

is the town council (Stadtverordnetenversammlung), which has at least eleven members, and according to population may have many more; in Berlin there are 225. These are elected for four years. The town's executive may be either the burgomaster or the *Magistrat*. The latter consists of paid members, who are officials, and of unpaid members. The paid members are appointed by the town council for twelve years. At least one-third of the Magistrat must be unpaid. Prussian municipalities have made great use of their general powers, especially in public health. Although rigidly restricted as regards education and police, in other matters they have greater power of initiative than the town councils in England. With them what is not prohibited can be done. In England, what they do must come within the limits laid down in public health and other enactments of the central legislature. These German municipalities appear to have unlimited power to buy and hold or resell land within and without their borders—a most important matter in town-planning. In England such powers are only recently being given and used.

The general picture is one of a rigid local bureaucratic system run by local officials, but held in by the power of the purse in taxation, which remains in the hands of the elected council. In the larger towns, on the other hand, municipal adventures, such as social "activities" and activities in trading and in various other directions, are very striking.

BERLIN

The administrative machinery of Berlin may be briefly outlined. In 1920 by law 94 local authorities, including 59 rural communes, were incorporated with Berlin under a special federation (Zweckverband) giving unified local government. The Greater Berlin thus constituted has an area of about 320 square miles and a population of about 4 millions.

The unified government for local purposes is administered by the *town council* (Stadtverordnetenversammlung), consisting of 225 members, elected by adult suffrage for four years.

The council appoints an executive (*Magistrat*) of not more than thirty members, some paid, but at least twelve unpaid.

Berlin is divided for administrative work into twenty districts (*Bezirke*) and the same number of *district councils*, each comprising the district representatives of the town council and, in addition, from fifteen to forty-five further directly elected members.

Each district council has an executive *Bezirksamt* comprising seven members.

These district councils have much local power over local administration, subject to following the lines laid down for the whole city.

It will be seen that, although the greater local authorities have an increasing measure of autonomy, local administration is also largely under central control. Paid and unpaid officials of local authorities have much power independent of local elected representatives of the people.

Throughout Germany the control of its system of compulsory school education is chiefly central, but the cost is local.

The poor law system in towns forms part of the work of the German municipalities, as will be the case in Great Britain from 1930 onwards. Each German municipality can work out its own plans, free from outside State interference, as in the running of its gas or electricity works. Education also is administered locally, but subject to rigid national control. Disputes between towns and country districts, or between two of the latter, are settled locally, or referred to the Federal Settlement Board. The standard of relief of the poor is low in many rural districts. In towns it may be high, and it is not bound down by restrictions which prevent its having a preventive character. What is known as the Elberfeld system has not succeeded in the large towns, owing to the difficulty in securing the services of satisfactory citizens to undertake the localised individual supervision.

Medical relief to the poor was formerly given, as in England, by specially appointed doctors; but, as in France, this has been partly replaced by "free choice of doctor", insurance doctors being called on for the work, and payment being made on the basis of an official minimum scale. In Berlin the majority of doctors for the poor are specially appointed doctors.

PUBLIC HOSPITAL SYSTEM

Most German hospitals are supported out of public funds, if insurance funds also be regarded as such. The communes must provide hospital treatment for the poor when this is required. In earlier decades the public hospitals provided by communes and municipalities were exclusively for the destitute sick, but their use and their quality has extended to other classes.

W. H. Dawson (*Municipal Life, etc., in Germany*, 1914) gives the total number of public hospitals in Germany in 1885 as 1,706, with 75,000 beds. In 1927 hospitals had increased to 2,964, and beds to 314,019. This was accompanied by a great increase in private hospitals, for the provision of which permission of the State authority is required. There are now 833 private hospitals, with 44,310 beds. All hospitals are subject to State supervision, and the hospitals connected with Universities are State institutions.

German Universities in the main are State institutions, though Cologne and Hamburg Universities are largely municipal. Although they are State supported, freedom in teaching and research is maintained by statute. All appointments, including those of the Medical Faculty, are made by the University, and the professor is in complete control of teaching facilities. He is, nevertheless, a State official. Even in municipal hospitals and clinics the same freedom of medical teaching in the main is found. Most professors and clinical teachers are almost completely divorced from private medical practice; they are seldom in touch with the doctors of the community.

Larger municipalities have provided, in addition, children's and other special hospitals, sanatoria, dispensaries, convalescent homes, etc. The provision of communal hospitals for infectious diseases is obligatory under an Imperial law dated 1900.

In Berlin there are three classes of hospitals: municipal hospitals, with some 16,000 beds (March 1929); voluntary hospitals—Jewish, Catholic, Evangelical, and private sanatoria; and State hospitals attached to the University of Berlin. The private hospitals and the University hospitals between them have about 12,000 beds, without counting beds for mental and infectious cases and for the aged.

The municipality bears the cost of the poor patients, including patients from welfare institutions, but may charge according to means. There is an approximate upper limit of earnings of 3,000 marks a year for welfare patients. About 65 per cent. of patients in the public hospitals are sent from the insurance funds, who pay a fixed charge to the hospital authorities, which at present is 6·80 marks a day, the *per capita* cost being 11 marks. This inadequate payment for hospital treatment is a general feature of the Continental experience of sick funds. At present there is incomplete, sometimes overlapping, hospital provision by—

> The Sick Funds of Insurance Organisations,
> Municipalities and other Public Authorities,
> Private Welfare Institutions;

and the insurance problem in Germany is further complicated by the fact that the sick and disabled are medically provided for, with very unsatisfactory co-ordination, both by sick funds and by the Invalidity Organisation (Landesversicherungsanstalten). In order to help co-ordination, the Reich Labour Ministry has recently published Model Regulations (especially for tuberculosis and venereal diseases), prescribing methods of co-operation for the bodies concerned (February 27, 1929).

SOCIAL WELFARE WORK (SOCIALE FÜRSORGE)

The public (not insurance) services for the treatment of sickness are becoming unified with those of health welfare work in Germany; but the municipal health office and the child welfare office are related to an extent which varies greatly according to local conditions, personal and other. Four partners are concerned in health work: the *State*, which legislates and may initiate administration; the *communes*, legally competent to administer health work; the *sickness funds*, which are vitally concerned in health work; and *private welfare organisations*. The part borne by each of these varies locally; but, except in the large towns, the activities of sickness funds overshadow the three others.

As already explained, in public health work each commune is a law unto itself, the chief federal or State legislation being restricted to infectious diseases, venereal diseases, and tuberculosis. For those in need, the Reich Welfare Law of February 1924 substituted District and State Welfare Associations for the old poor relief. These also carry on maternity and child welfare work for those in need of help. In Prussia the chief measure concerning infectious diseases is the law of 1905, amended in 1926.

The help of these welfare associations is conditional on the need for extraneous help, and their work does not as a rule include preventive measures. The relief granted, however, now extends beyond the bare minimum of existence.

It is becoming increasingly recognised that it is unpractical to continue to work various agencies of health work in watertight compartments; and that private welfare associations, communal authorities, and sickness funds may advantageously form joint associations for this work. The social help given by the sickness funds is described on pages 147 *et seq.* The social help to the destitute and in hospitals has already been indicated. There remains the social help given in maternity and child welfare organisations, in school medical and welfare work, in tuberculosis work, and for venereal diseases, on which further particulars may be given.

At this point we may indicate some of the subsidies for health, insurance, and welfare work which are given by the Reich Government.

The following figures for 1928 are extracted from the *International Health Year Book* (1928) of the League of Nations.

GERMAN BUDGET FOR 1928

	Marks
To encourage sanitary improvement, especially for the protection of the young and infirm, and to secure diffusion of hygienic knowledge	500,000
To the struggle against alcoholism and the diseases favoured by it (tuberculosis and venereal), and to the protection of mentally affected	1,400,000
For medical research	200,000
To the expense of an institute concerned with the struggle against infant mortality	240,000
Specific scientific researches	3,000,000
Complementary contributions to invalidity insurance societies (1927)	209,800,000
Maternity assistance to wives and daughters of insured persons	30,000,000
State institutions for the destitute	1,432,000

These are only a few of the total items of subsidies granted by the Reich.

MATERNITY SERVICES

Large subsidies (in 1928 the amount was 30 million marks) are given by the Reich for assistance under local schemes to women in child-bed. Puerperal mortality is high, notwithstanding the benefits under the national insurance Acts. In Berlin in 1926 the number of deaths registered as caused by puerperal sepsis (Kindbettfieber) was 299, the registered births for the same year being 46,704. This means a total death-rate in that year from puerperal sepsis of 6·40 per 1,000 births—a terrible figure. Over three-fourths of this mortality from sepsis was associated with abortions —another terrible figure.

The Berlin birth-rate (live-births) in the same year was

only 11·6 per 1,000 of population, and of the births over 19 per cent. were illegitimate.

Dr. Roesle is of the opinion that "abortions are perhaps as numerous as normal births". A large number of these must be intentional.

All midwives are required to possess a diploma of competency.

In Prussia and some other States an eighteen months' course of training is required for midwives; in Bavaria and Saxony a course of twelve months; and in some smaller States of nine months.

In Prussia nearly 90 per cent. of births are attended by midwives. Even in Berlin, where there are over 1,000 midwives, three-fourths of the midwives are in private practice, and only one-fourth in hospitals.

In areas in which, owing to unfavourable conditions, the midwifery service is inadequate, action has occasionally been taken by local authorities to subsidise midwives. Repetition courses for midwives have also been initiated in some States, attendance at these being required at varying intervals of three to ten years. The general status of midwives in Germany is, however, unsatisfactory. They are badly paid and have no pensions.

In Berlin no midwives are engaged in practice on behalf of the town council, and there are no arrangements for the public guarantee of the doctor's fee when called in by a midwife for a complicated case.

Nearly 60 per cent. of all births in Berlin occur in hospitals. For care of these, if parents are insured, the insurance societies pay; about 10 per cent. pay for themselves; for the rest the municipality is responsible.

Antenatal care is supplied to some extent by the city, at the University clinics, and by the insurance funds. In Berlin there are forty-three Pregnancy Consultation Centres and fifteen Marriage Consultation Centres.

Maternity Work through Insurance.—Details are given in *Compulsory Sickness Insurance*, 1927, and in *Benefits of the German Sickness System*, by Drs. Goldmann and Grotjahn (both issued by the International Labour Office, 1928). A brief outline only is needed here.

The number of women who have to bear the triple burden and responsibility of maternity, domestic work, and industrial employment has increased in Germany as elsewhere; and associated with this has been a marked increase in the proportion of miscarriages to live-births in women workers (see also p. 142). The figures supplied by various insurance societies in this respect are appalling, especially in view of the serious after-consequences in many cases of miscarriage and abortion, whether intentionally caused or not.

As the result of successive insurance enactments, maternal and child welfare have been consolidated, making insurance funds responsible for protection of maternity in insured women and in the dependents of insured men; while district welfare associations are responsible for aid to persons of small means who have no claims on the insurance funds. As already seen, the Reich gives large subsidies for these purposes (p. 142). The Reich contributes 50 marks towards the maternity benefit of dependents for each confinement. The sickness fund is responsible for the cost of this benefit only for personally insured women.

The statutory insurance benefits are :—

1. Attendance of a midwife, drugs, and appliances, and such medical treatment as may be needed.
2. An allowance of 10 marks towards the expense of confinement.
3. A daily cash benefit equal to that for sickness benefit for four weeks before and six weeks after confinement. It is payable for two additional weeks if the insured woman abstains from all remunerative work during that period.
4. So long as the insured woman nurses her infant, she is entitled to a nursing bonus, equal to half the sickness benefit, until the end of the twelfth week.

The sick fund may give treatment and maintenance in a maternity home, or attendance by a nurse, in entire or partial substitution for the maternity cash benefit.

Maternity benefit is also granted to the wife, daughters,

step-daughters, and adopted daughters of an insured person who are members of his household.

The cash benefit is inadequate, thus tempting women to work too long before and too soon after confinements; it is regrettable, therefore, that very few sickness funds have exceeded the legal minimum.

An employer must not employ a worker for six weeks after confinement, and notice of dismissal during six weeks before or after confinement is invalid.

There is a strong feeling in some quarters that it should be made compulsory on women entitled to benefit from sick funds to consult the maternity and child welfare centres set up by municipalities or voluntary organisations. Already there is growing up co-operation between the funds and the centres. Thus in Leipzig the local sickness funds bore about 11 per cent. of the running expenses of the welfare centres of the city in the year 1925.

Similarly I found that in Berlin the Association of Sick Funds arranged for antenatal consultations in the forty-three welfare centres, and for marriage consultations in fifteen centres. The Erfurt General Local Sickness Fund maintains its own welfare centre, at which over 68 per cent. of all women confined in 1925 received advice during pregnancy.

In some cities sickness funds bear the cost of providing a woman to do household work during the lying-in period.

CHILD WELFARE WORK

In 1924, the year in which the Social Aid Decree was passed, the Federal Child Welfare Act was also enacted. This Act included a preamble to the effect that "every German child is entitled to education with a view to its physical, mental, and moral well-being". This was a normal sequence of the formal constitution of the German Reich (August 1919), which laid special emphasis on the duty of State and local authorities to take steps for the preservation of the family as a whole, and for its physical and social amelioration. Under a special measure of the Reich (*Reichsgrundsätze*), which deals with the conditions of relief, it is laid down that relief must be given on the case method and based on a study of individual needs.

There are now *infant welfare institutions* throughout Germany, controlled by the communes or by private welfare organisations. In 1926 these numbered over 5,000.

In Prussia and some other States the special training of welfare doctors is regulated, but this is not compulsory; welfare nurses must have a three-years' training for this work, after which a special diploma is given.

The arrangements of welfare institutions are supervised by the public medical officers or communal doctors. These doctors also engage in private medical practice. I was informed that no considerable difficulty had arisen as to possible interference with private practice. Some treatment is given at the Berlin centres, as of syphilis and of minor ailments.

In Berlin there are eighty-four infant consultation centres, with ninety-nine doctors and a number of nurses. At each of these one or more doctors attend for two to three hours. Each doctor receives a monthly salary, related to the number of hours of work. There are 191 nurses connected with the infant and antenatal consultation centres.

Milk mixtures are provided when medically ordered, not for ordinary nursing. Owing to the current dispute as to venereal disease centres (May 1929), the associated doctors have announced that they will forbid doctors to attend infant consultations for treatment. No general objection is made to the home visits of a Fürsorgerin; but it is alleged that occasionally such visits lead to withdrawal of children from private practice to institutions.

At these consultation centres in most parts of Germany, as a rule, treatment is not given.

In addition to the centres, there are in towns also in-patient children's hospitals, clinics, crèches, etc., which need not be specially described. The best known is the Kaiserin-Auguste-Viktoria-Haus at Charlottenberg, Berlin. This comprises in-patient departments, a training department for nurses, and other activities.

Child Welfare Work through Insurance.—The mothers of over 65 per cent. of the total children born in Germany are beneficiaries of insurance funds; and the insurance benefits in maternity (midwife, medical care, domestic assistance, a financial grant) may properly be regarded as important items of child welfare work. The continuance of this work at welfare centres is most desirable; and the Federal Insurance Code of October 1926 emphasises this in a clause which states that each sickness fund when granting nursing benefits may

draw attention to the advantage of making use of maternity and infant welfare centres or similar institutions.

In accordance with this, some sickness funds have made the payment of nursing benefit conditional on the production of a certificate from the local welfare centre. In a few places, as at Düsseldorf, payments of maternity benefits in cash are made at the welfare centre by a woman official of the sickness fund.[1]

In Erfurt the general local sickness fund has its own infant welfare centre. This is undesirable; it implies two centres, one for insured and one for non-insured, and is wasteful of working power.

The sickness funds in most of Germany have, however, contributed very little to the support of infant welfare centres. It is unnecessary to emphasise the intimate relation between child defects and diseases and claims on insurance funds in subsequent life.

School Medical Work

Germany was a pioneer in the application of hygiene to school life, and some of the most important advances in school hygiene have been made by German school doctors. The first school doctor was appointed in Wiesbaden in 1895, others slowly following this example. There was much opposition to the work for some years. School sisters were initiated in 1908.

Drs. Goldmann and Grotjahn's report, p. 90.

School work is very largely subsidised from State funds in each German State, and the organisation is largely regulated by the State.

In Prussia the Kreis medical officers give assistance in the examination of building projects, and the local medical officers of health supervise the school-children. More exact medical inspection has gradually been introduced in the larger towns, special school doctors being appointed for this purpose. The completeness of this service varies greatly in different towns in each State; and in rural districts the service may be rudimentary. As a rule no treatment is provided by the school medical service for defects found in medical inspection.

In Berlin, as in other cities, school medical work forms a division of public health administration. Its position is shown in the following scheme. First, there is the primary division into

Public Health Work, and
Welfare and Youth Work,

the last including care of the destitute. Under Public Health Work are included the following sub-divisions:—

Epidemiology—including investigations, disinfection, vaccination, baths, etc.,
School hygiene,
Social hygiene,
Hospitals and asylums,
Ambulances and first aid,
Financial,
Legal.

There are seventy-nine whole-time and twelve part-time school doctors in Berlin, some of them qualified as medical officers of health. The part-time school doctors may engage in private practice. Prior to the appointment of these whole-time officers, the medical school service for twenty-five years had been in the hands of private physicians. On behalf of the medical profession the objection to giving school medical work to whole-time medical officers was strongly maintained, and the G.B.M.A. (p. 163) intervened on behalf of the displaced officers, and succeeded in obtaining financial compensation for them if they were over fifty-five years old. This was made conditional on their holding themselves ready in case of recall.

The aim is to have one school doctor to 400 to 500 scholars. Each school doctor has two whole-time school nurses to help him. In 1927 there were 842 schools in Berlin and some 385,000 scholars.

The school doctor is required to examine each scholar once in two years. Treatment of defects, except dental, is very limited. Nurses care for minor skin ailments, etc. Children are sent in large numbers to sanatoria and to holiday homes. When such defects as adenoids are discovered, the parent is referred to a private doctor, or sent to one of the polyclinics.

Polyclinics in Berlin may belong to sickness funds. They may also be private organisations, and there are more than a hundred of the latter. These private polyclinics sometimes contract with sick funds for the treatment of special cases.

There is one special ophthalmic doctor for the schools, evidently an inadequate provision. Eye defects found by school doctors are referred to the private doctor, or to the sickness funds or welfare associations, the decision on this point resting with the school nurse. Among the school doctors there is also a specialist for ear diseases, and one for nervous diseases.

In Berlin eighteen school dental clinics are maintained, three or four dentists being engaged for each clinic. There are thirty-five whole-time and twenty part-time dentists attached to the clinics, as well as a considerable number of nurses. Every child is examined each second year, and it is hoped to reduce the interval to one year. All defects are treated, and there is no reference to private dentists. No objection was raised at first; but private dentists now protest because the municipality has begun to treat adults for dental disease.

The school dental clinics are closed at 3 p.m., and may be used later in the day for welfare patients if not otherwise fully occupied. Here again in Berlin, which is noted for its socialist policy, no poverty test is imposed.

SCHOOL MEDICAL WORK THROUGH INSURANCE

Some large sickness funds contribute towards social help by municipalities for school children, especially in providing sanatoria or convalescent home treatment. In other instances they provide independently convalescent homes and institutional beds for the accommodation of children. On a more limited scale, some sickness funds have made provision for proper feeding of the children of insured persons (Ernährungsfürsorge). Goldmann and Grotjahn state that in 1925, 45 per cent. of the cost of school meals provided by the municipality of Cologne was defrayed by the Cologne sickness funds. Certain sickness funds have also contributed largely to the arrangements for ortho-pædic gymnastics for scholars.

In view of the important gain to insurance funds when children leave school with sound teeth, it is not surprising that in this field sickness funds have actively contributed to municipal school dentists; while others provide facilities for the treatment of school children in their own dental clinics.

It may be said that in smaller towns and rural districts activities of sickness funds, and that in large cities activities of municipal authorities, predominate in the directions indicated above.

The present position in regard to school children, as also for infants, and for the treatment of disease, especially of tuberculosis and venereal diseases, is one which calls for action directed towards pooling the arrangements made by communal authorities and by sickness funds.

TUBERCULOSIS

In Germany the control of tuberculosis has been entrusted for many years to the German *Central Committee*

for the Prevention of Tuberculosis (Central Komité zür Be-
kämpfung der Tuberkulose). A variety of societies has been
combined under the wing of this society. Although a
private body, this committee has a semi-official character.
Its governing body, or *Präsidium*, consists of:—

The Presidents of
{
Reich Health Office,
Reich Insurance Office,
Reich Insurance Association for Em-
ployees;
}

A representative of
{
Reich Ministry of the Interior,
Prussian Ministry for Public Welfare,
Prussian Ministry for Science, Art, and
Education;
}
and a number of leading physicians.

This Präsidium has an advisory committee, consisting,
among others, of tuberculosis physicians, or representatives of provinces and administrative districts, and of
directors of provincial insurance societies and sick funds.

Funds are derived mainly from contributions from the
Reich, among which is the product of the alcohol monopoly
fund; and in Prussia funds come also from lotteries authorised by the State.[1]

The work of the Central Committee is partly educational,
and partly concerned with the provision of sanatoria, convalescent homes, and other institutions, which may all be
regarded as preventoriums.

In 1928 there were in Germany 193 sanatoria for adult
patients, having 204,260 beds; and 382 sanatoria, with
30,678 beds, for children with pulmonary and non-pul-
monary tuberculosis, or threatened with it. In addition,
there were 196 forest recreation establishments and schools,
31 convalescent homes, with 1,463 beds, and 339 tuberculosis
hospitals or wards in general hospitals.

In 1922 there were in Germany some 2,000 *tuberculosis
welfare institutes* or dispensaries. Treatment is not given at
these. They are diagnostic centres and centres for social
work.

[1] For further particulars on this and other administrative details see Dr. G.
Frey's *Public Health Service in Germany* (League of Nations publication).

There is no legal regulation of the struggle against tuberculosis applicable to the whole of Germany. In some States there is compulsory notification of open cases of tuberculosis, but not in all. Similarly, municipal arrangements for the control of tuberculosis are very unequal and need further development and unification. The insurance sickness and invalidity associations do a vast amount of anti-tuberculosis work, which is outlined below.

Many sickness funds pay for the consultation work done in tuberculosis institutes. Tuberculosis is a disease which often causes disability after the benefits of sickness insurance have been exhausted; and there is great need for unification of action as to tuberculosis between sickness and invalidity insurance organisations, to avoid delay in treatment and to secure maximum economic efficiency.

Tuberculosis Work and Insurance.—In England a special sanatorium benefit was initiated in the Health Insurance Act of 1912. Soon, however, the absurdity of attempting to separate the campaign against tuberculosis—a communicable disease—into two compartments, for the insured and the non-insured, became obvious, and anti-tuberculosis work was transferred entirely to public health authorities. By them institutional treatment is nearly always given gratuitously to all needing it. In Germany a dual, if not a triple, organisation continues: for the non-insured, tuberculosis work is inadequate; and for the insured, there is an unfortunate tendency to transfer the burden of needed help from sickness to invalidity funds.

The long duration of pulmonary tuberculosis lends itself to this; many insured persons exhaust their sickness benefit and continue ill. Hitherto invalidity insurance funds have done much more anti-tuberculosis work than sickness funds; but now early examinations, including the use of X-ray examinations, are being encouraged, though still not adequately, and very inadequately for the dependents of the insured. This work is being aided by the employment of health visitors by sickness funds to help in discovering cases and to arrange for examinations. This is done at tuberculosis centres (Fürsorgestellen), where expert help is available. Sickness funds are urged by official circulars from the Reich to aid in establishing and maintaining these centres. The extent of their contributions to this end varies greatly, but the movement is extending. Occasionally sickness funds maintain tuberculosis consultation centres of their own; and in Berlin two centres of this character are also subsidised by the municipality, so that they may be available for the general public.

As regards sanatorium or hospital treatment, it is evident that restrictions dependent on the financial reserves of a given sickness fund must tend to minimise effectiveness of action. The position in Germany, notwithstanding the vast expenditure on sanatoria, etc., cannot be regarded as satisfactory. Nor is the position as regards home treatment of insured tuberculous patients satisfactory. Home treatment is indispensable, especially in view of the deficiency of sanatorium beds. But it was pointed out to me by those responsible for large sickness insurance funds that the capitation payment to doctors is not in the consumptive's interests, as in practice it sometimes means relative neglect of the patient.

VENEREAL DISEASES

By the Prussian Epidemic Law of 1905, professional prostitutes, if diseased or suspected of being diseased, could be subjected to observation, and to isolation if found diseased. Similar enactments were made in other German States. This law was found to touch only a small part of the total evil; and compulsory examination of prostitutes was abandoned two years ago.

In December 1918 the Reich Government made it obligatory on all persons suffering from venereal diseases to secure treatment; doctors were made responsible for instructing their patients, and were obliged to give each patient a printed paper of instructions at the beginning and at the end of treatment.

For a short period the Reich Government gave subsidies

for the provision of consultation centres (Beratungstellen), to which skilled doctors were attached for each special district. Communes, sickness funds, and State insurance associations also gave financial support to these.

At the end of 1922 there were 180 such consultation centres. Treatment was not given at these centres.

In 1920 the Reich Insurance Office empowered sickness funds to make it a duty under their health regulations that all cases of venereal disease in their members and the families of these should be compulsorily notified.

The Act passed by the Reichstag in January 1927 has codified and extended previous enactments. It requires that all persons "knowingly suffering from contagious venereal disease or having reasonable cause to believe themselves infected, shall submit themselves to medical treatment".

The competent sanitary authority may require persons whom they reasonably believe to be suffering from and disseminating venereal disease to produce a medical certificate of health.

Suspected persons may be compelled, if diagnosis is confirmed, to undergo treatment or be sent into a hospital. When compulsory treatment is enforced, this does not extend to the administration of mercury, arsenical preparations, or to the examination of cerebro-spinal fluid except with the patient's consent. Blood examinations may be made without the patient's consent.

Any person knowingly suffering from contagious venereal disease, or having reasonable cause to believe himself infected, is liable to three years' imprisonment if he marries without informing the other party to the marriage of such infection. This applies also to cohabitation without marriage.

Only those persons authorised to practise medicine in Germany are permitted to treat venereal diseases and diseases of the genital organs. Absentee treatment—that is, otherwise than on personal diagnosis—and the giving of advice verbally or otherwise for self-treatment are prohibited.

Every person treating a venereally diseased person is

required to instruct him as to the character of the disease and the danger of contagion, and to furnish the patient with an officially authorised memorandum.

If a person under treatment eludes such treatment, or if he otherwise, in consequence of his vocation or personal circumstances, especially endangers other persons, the physician in charge of the case is required to notify the sanitary authority, or at the option of the supreme State Authority to notify a venereal disease advisory bureau.

Advertisement of supposed anti-venereal remedies is prohibited.

To Dr. Breger (*Oberregierungsrat im Reichsgesundheitsamt*) I am indebted for much of the information which follows.

There has been no general adoption of a system of gratuitous treatment of venereal disease, such as exists in England. This is regarded as unnecessary, inasmuch as 80 per cent. of the population is insured for medical attendance, either for sickness or invalidity.

For the poor each commune must pay if there is no insurance.

Attempts are now being made to secure an approach to unification of the communal anti-venereal work, sickness insurance anti-venereal work, and invalidity insurance anti-venereal work.

In this disease, as in tuberculosis, there is a tendency to shunt responsibility from the sickness to the invalidity insurance funds. Obviously this is short-sighted and detrimental to the funds as well as to the patients, as only early treatment systematically continued can secure the prevention of protracted sickness.

In Berlin there is (June 1929) an acute dispute between the municipality of Berlin and the medical profession, centring on the treatment of venereal diseases. In this city some treatment of venereal patients is given at certain centres, and it is in connection with the proposed extension of treatment to other centres that the present fight has arisen. The organised doctors have decided not only to withdraw their members from working at these centres, but also from the child welfare centres (at which there is little or no treatment), unless they receive an undertaking that municipal treatment will not be undertaken at the proposed additional consultation centres.

I visited one of these centres (Beratungs Anstalt), formed under the invalidity insurance system and subsidised by the city, and from its chief, Dr. Citron, received the following information. Any person can come to the centre for advice without payment; but he is then referred to an approved doctor after examination. This may be one of the insurance ambulatories, a polyclinic, or a hospital. The patient is sent with a report, which is stamped by the prospective doctor, who is expected to return it to the consultation centre. Patients rarely fail to go on for treatment. A similar arrangement holds good throughout Germany.

No regulation compels patients to attend the consultation centre; but they come, as Dr. Citron explained, because they get good independent advice and no money obligation is incurred.

There is a welfare institution specially concerned with venereal diseases of children. This is staffed by women doctors and teachers, who make family inquiries where these are indicated.

At Dr. Citron's centre 53,000 men and 12,000 women have been advised in eleven years, the average cost per consultation being 2 marks.

The friction already mentioned has arisen in connection with the new law on venereal diseases, which, in substituting sanitary for police control of venereal diseases, has rendered it necessary to arrange for the treatment of the poor and other non-insured persons. In Berlin temporary arrangements have been made for the doctors of the poor to treat such patients in their own consulting-rooms at the expense of the city.

The municipality has ten consultation centres, at which —unlike in Dr. Citron's centre—treatment of venereal diseases is given, as well as ten centres, of which Dr. Citron's is one, at which no treatment is given. This has been tolerated by the medical profession; but there is strong objection to multiplication of these centres. The opposition is organised through the Gross-Berliner Ärztebund, acting for the doctors, and since May 12, 1929, doctors have been withdrawn from these and from child welfare centres until the municipality consents not to extend treatment at the centres.

Behind this current instance of strenuous struggle between the municipality of Berlin and the syndicated doctors of the city is the apprehension that the loss of opportunity to treat venereal disease in private practice will go far to destroy the relatively small amount of private medical practice remaining outside sickness insurance. Already the sickness insurance funds cover a majority of the population for sickness, including such specialist treatment as is required for venereal diseases.

Under the system of capitation fees for medical attendance now commonly adopted by many funds, there is risk of superficial and unsatisfactory treatment of diseases like syphilis and gonorrhœa. In many sickness funds only a fraction of the cost of drugs is paid by the funds in the case of dependents,[1] and this again may mean unsatisfactory and incomplete treatment. There appears also to be fear in the mind of some of the insured that certification of venereal disease under insurance will give rise to economic or other difficulties.

As in tuberculosis, though to a less degree, there is risk of a hiatus rather than of overlapping between invalidity and sickness insurance funds in the treatment of venereal diseases.

In some districts various insurance funds have combined to secure skilled treatment for venereal diseases in special institutions at the expense of the funds; and this is a vast improvement on the system which leaves the treatment of these diseases in the hands of individual insurance doctors.

[1] Goldmann and Grotjahn, *op. cit.*, p. 141.

It would be better still if these institutions were run by local authorities, so that the non-insured might also benefit. In Frankfort-on-Main the municipality does combine with the insurance funds for this purpose.

SICKNESS AND INVALIDITY INSURANCE

Although the chief facts concerning German insurance are to be found in various accessible publications, it is necessary to summarise them briefly here, as otherwise it is difficult to appreciate at their full value the persistent discussions and disputations and the underlying seething dissatisfaction which exists. This dissatisfaction appears to be shared by insurance societies (sick funds) and the medical practitioners of Germany alike, although it is much more keenly felt by the medical profession, who freely express themselves as in bondage. Private medical practice has become, for most of them, a shadow of the private practice of the past.

Details of the working of German sickness insurance are given in *Compulsory Sickness Insurance*, 1927, and in *Benefits of the German Sickness Insurance System*, by Drs. Goldmann and Grotjahn, both published by the International Labour Office of the League of Nations. Only a brief summary is given here; but further particulars based on personal inquiries are added.

The first Act on sickness insurance was passed by the German Reichstag in 1883. In subsequent years the number of classes insured was steadily increased and benefits were enlarged.

In 1911 the Acts relating to insurance against sickness, invalidity and accident were incorporated in a single Federal Insurance Code, and provision for surviving dependents was for the first time introduced. Miners and salaried employees retained separate systems of insurance.

Under these various enactments the executive work of sickness insurance was entrusted to legally authorised sickness funds or societies. These are autonomous, and have a large measure of freedom in the granting of benefits, the State confining itself to supervision and safeguarding of the efficiency of the funds. This supervision is carried out by officials, who act as courts of supervision, arbitration, and appeal.

They are:—

Insurance Offices (Versicherungsämter),
Upper Insurance Offices (Oberversicherungsämter),
Federal Insurance Office (Reichsversicherungsamt).

Sickness funds may be either on a local or an occupational basis. A large number of the smaller funds have been abolished. In 1925 the total funds numbered 7,670, not much more than one-third of their number in 1885.

The local Insurance Funds in 1925 had 67·6 per cent.,
Works Funds had 18·7 per cent.,
Rural Societies had 11·3 per cent.,
Guilds had 2·4 per cent.,

of the total insured population in their respective organisations.[1]

Sickness insurance applies only to persons engaged in a paid employment; no maximum limit of earnings is laid down for industrial employees. For salaried employees and officials (Angestelle) the maximum limit is an income of 6,000 marks per annum. (A mark is nearly equivalent to an English penny or two cents.)

Persons engaged in home industry (Hausgewerbetreibende) are also included in the general compulsion.

At its beginning German Sickness Insurance included less than 10 per cent. of the population; in 1914 this proportion had increased to 23 per cent.; in 1928 it had become about 33 per cent. of the total population. Of the total occupied population 63 per cent., and of the wage-earning population 77 per cent., were compulsorily insured in 1925.

The grant of sickness benefits to family dependents is left to the discretion of individual sickness funds. It is estimated that not much less than 19 or 20 million family dependents are now potential or actual recipients of medical benefits,

[1] Goldmann and Grotjahn, *op. cit.*, p. 8.

making a total of three-fifths of Germany's total population. To this must be added four millions who are insured in "middle-class" funds on the principle of mutual aid.

The following table extracted from the above-cited source shows the progress of actual membership of the legal sickness funds :—

	Total Members	Percentage of Female to Male Members
1885	4,294,173	22·2
1895	7,525,524	29·0
1905	11,184,476	33·9
1915	13,840,848	76·2
1925	18,234,970[1]	61·6

[1] Not including 817,845 members of miners' benefit societies, and 1,122,541 members of substitute sickness societies, i.e. friendly societies based on the principle of mutual aid.

The contribution payable must not exceed 7·5 per cent. of the basic wage of each class of worker. Of this, two-thirds is payable by the insured person and one-third by the employer.

In guild funds the contribution may be equally shared between employer and employed.

In miners' funds the relative contributions of insured and employer are three-fifths and two-fifths.

Benefits are monetary and in kind. The chief cash benefit is one-half of the basic wage, payable from the fourth day of sickness, or the day of incapacity for work, if this is later than the fourth day.

The maternity benefit includes sick pay for two weeks and a lump sum of 10 marks.

The *Sick Benefit* includes a cash payment for twenty-six weeks of at least one-half the worker's basic wage. It also comprises medical treatment, including the supply of medicines and appliances (spectacles, trusses, etc.), and hospital treatment. During hospital treatment half the sick pay is given. The limitation of medical attendance to six months will be noted. Sick funds may give additional benefits if their finance permits.

In 1925, in funds subject to the Federal Insurance Code,[1] there were 54·8 cases of sickness among men and 46 cases among women per 100 insured of each sex.

In the same year, among sick men the average duration of sick benefit was 22·5 days, and among sick women 28 days, while the number of days of sickness per insured person was 12·5.

The Maternity Benefit, in addition to the monetary allowance mentioned above, provides medical treatment, the services of a midwife, and medicine and appliances. A lump sum of 10 marks is given towards the expenses of confinement; and there is also a nursing bonus, equal to half the sickness benefit, continued until the end of the twelfth week after confinement if the insured nurses her child.

Treatment in a maternity home may replace the maternity cash benefit, or half this cash benefit may be deducted to provide attendance by home nurses.

Family Maternity Benefit is extended to the wife and daughters of an insured man if domiciled with him. The rules of the fund may include a clause requiring them to draw the attention of the recipients of nursing benefit (during lactation) to welfare centres for advice for mothers and infants.

A Funeral Benefit is given, in general amounting to twenty times the daily basic wage.

Family Medical Benefit is an optional benefit; but the great majority of sickness funds now include this in the benefit for the insured. Perhaps even more important than this is the increasing realisation that limitation of medical treatment to twenty-six weeks may be serious for insured patients. A few funds have extended medical benefit to one year, and perhaps one-eighth of all funds have extended it to thirty-nine weeks.

The medical arrangements include the services of specialists as well as of general practitioners. About four-

[1] *Compulsory Sickness Insurance* (League of Nations Publications, 1927).

fifths of the entire German medical profession work for
the sick funds, and for the majority of these, insurance
work is the chief source of their livelihood. Only about
5 per cent. of German medical practitioners are engaged in
private practice alone. There appears to be every reason to
think that sickness insurance provides more than half of
the total incomes derived from medical practice in Germany.

Payment of doctors may be by any of the following
methods :—

1. Payment by attendance.
2. A capitation fee per insured person whom the doctor
   engages to treat. In England this is known as the
   "panel" system.
3. The same as 2, except that the capitation payments are
   made into a pooled fund, from which doctors are paid
   according to their actual attendances.
4. Payment per case of sickness attended.
5. Payment by fixed salaries.
6. Whole-time doctors.

Medical attendance in the German system includes hospital
and expert medical services, in addition to the care given
by a family doctor.

Each of the methods of payment of doctors enumerated
above has been tried by various funds; but with the
increasing medical pressure secured by combined bargaining
of medical associations (see p. 166), free choice of doctors
has mostly won the day, the majority of funds having
unwillingly yielded this point, so far as home visits and
attendance at the doctor's surgery are concerned.

At this point it is convenient to consider this and allied
problems from the point of view of the *Medical Profession
in Germany*. According to recent statistics, there are 48,507
medical men and women living in Germany, of whom
2,376 are women. Of these more than a fourth describe
themselves as specialists. In the large cities the number of
medical men is 1 to 806 of population, as against 1 to 1,820
in the small towns and rural districts.

In Berlin in 1929 there were 5,827 medical practitioners,

of whom 450 were officials. In 1927 the official figures state that there were 11,855 medical and dental students in the twenty-three German Universities.

The conditions of medical practice are determined in the main by the national system of sickness insurance; but the vast increase of hospital treatment of disease, the growth of school medicine, of maternity and child welfare work, and of treatment of tuberculosis and venereal disease, under the insurance system or through the collateral activities of public health authorities, have all acted in the same direction and made the German doctor more and more an official, and increasingly dependent for his livelihood on the insurance *caisses* or on the public authorities.

Medical Organisation

In Prussia there is a statutory *Medical Chamber* in each province. In Greater Berlin there is such a chamber, formed by the appointment of one member and one substitute for every fifty medical practitioners. The members number 109, and there is an equal number of substitutes.

This body deals with some matters of medical discipline. There is, in addition, a voluntary organisation, the *Greater Berlin Medical Association*, which conducts the economic struggle with insurance funds and official bodies. This, unlike the chamber, does not include the entire profession. It now has 4,400 members. Its general policy is one of retention of freedom of medical work.

The G.B.M.A. (Greater Berlin Medical Association) forms the local group of the chief economic organisation of the Leipzig Hartmann Association, as well as of the Central Professional Union of the German Medical Association.

About one-half of the Berlin medical profession, in addition, is organised in other professional societies.

Valuable details are given in *Krankenhilfe und Gesundheitsfürsorge durch die Ärzteschaft*, edited by Dr. med. Kurt Finkenrath, 1929. This contains contributions as to the medical politics of Greater Berlin by about twelve different physicians. Some of the following particulars are derived from this source.

The economic difficulties during the post-bellum failure of German finance meant chaos in medical contracts, and existent medical organisations were not strong enough to secure early reform.

In December 1918 a meeting was called at the instance of the Society for Reforming Abuses in Polyclinics, and it was decided that the urgent need of the moment was the foundation of a Medical Union for Greater Berlin.

Protracted discussion at this and subsequent meetings led to the formation of a new organisation with the declared objects of:—

1. Watching professional interests in economic, social, and ethical respects.
2. Promoting a fair distribution of all medical practitioners in the care of the sick.
3. Promoting the participation of medical practitioners in all questions of public health.
4. Promoting good fellowship amongst practitioners.

Local sub-groups were formed.

An early task of the new organisation was to consider proposed extensions of medical insurance (April 1920), and a resolution was adopted protesting against this "without any consultation with the medical profession or consideration for their necessities of life". There was a strong expression of opinion to the effect that the medical profession more and more was being given over to the control of the bureaucratism and fiscalism of the Krankenkassen (sickness funds), to the detriment of the health and welfare of the people. This conclusion was not reached without opposition; for the socialist practitioners proposed an unsuccessful resolution in amendment "welcoming the extension of compulsory medical insurance to further circles, as an advance in hygiene, as well as a step towards the socialisation of the whole medical profession".

The policy adopted by the G.B.M.A. was at once endorsed by the Central Union of Sick Fund Doctors of Berlin, and negotiations were begun in April 1920 with the associated sick funds, before whom the following requirements were placed:—

1. That all practitioners willing should be appointed for insurance work, free choice being allowed; and that any present insurance doctors who might suffer through this in their practice should be indemnified.
2. Adequate payment to be given to practitioners, up to the financial capacity of the sick funds.
3. Careful restriction of interference with the professional and personal freedom of the Kassen doctors.
4. Observance of Sunday rest by special arrangements.

Free choice of doctors was accepted by the sick funds, and suitable indemnification was accorded to doctors whose share of the sick fund medical work under the new arrangements was reduced.

During the rapid depreciation of the German mark in 1923 the G.B.M.A. declared all sick fund agreements to be suspended, and thenceforth the sick funds had to pay separately for each service rendered. No complete solution of the difficulties was found until the beginning of 1928. Prior to this, in 1924, the G.B.M.A. combined forces with the German Association of Medical Practitioners; and it was decided to unite the organisation of the G.B.M.A. and of the Berlin Division of the Hartmann Bund. This was accomplished in 1926, the G.B.M.A. being recognised as a provincial division of the Hartmann Bund.

In 1928 a contract for eight years was made by the G.B.M.A. with the Union of Krankenkassen of Greater Berlin and the Union of Managers of Krankenkassen of Berlin and neighbouring parts. This has been followed in some respects by satisfactory results.

The management of the insurance polyclinics has been investigated, and some steps taken to secure better co-operation with private physicians. Much charitable work in aid of impoverished doctors has been done.

The problem of middle-class compulsory sickness insurance has been investigated by the Hartmann Bund, along with a member of the G.B.M.A.

As to the activity of the G.B.M.A. respecting school doctors, see page 150, and respecting venereal diseases, see page 157. Some further items on this problem may be given here. In October 1927 the G.B.M.A. arranged with the Public Health Department of Berlin for a system of treatment of venereal diseases by physicians qualified for this work, on the principle of free choice of doctor. This was intended for poorer patients. In view of this it was agreed on January 1, 1928, that no further treatment centres for venereal diseases beyond the ten already belonging to the municipality should be begun by them without the consent of the G.B.M.A. The municipality now wishes to depart from this agreement (p. 155); but the medical profession, as voiced by the G.B.M.A., are not inclined to give way, though they wish heartily to support welfare centres, provided that treatment is completely separated from advice.

The general effect of the work of the G.B.M.A. has been to secure from the sickness funds uniform terms for physicians in Berlin on the basis of a free choice of doctor. It was also agreed that membership of the G.B.M.A. should be a condition of appointment as physician to a sickness fund. Before this was effected, each sick fund made its own arrangements with individual physicians as to conditions of medical work and remuneration.

The substitution of collective for individual bargaining has secured the admission of a much larger proportion of the total doctors into insurance practice.

Much difficulty has been experienced owing to different sickness funds varying the extent and character of medical attendance on dependents which is included in the sickness benefit.

Still greater difficulties arise in the working of the ambulatories or polyclinics for consultation and expert services. For these special doctors are appointed, and there is no free choice of doctor.

In Berlin recently there were 3,237 doctors engaged in sickness insurance work. Fresh appointments of doctors are only made as vacancies occur, and many doctors have to wait a long time before being admitted to the rank of doctors among whom "free choice of doctor" is allowed.

At an interview with Dr. Haedenkamp the following information was received.

Sickness funds are managed jointly by nominees of the workmen and masters, who together finance each fund. The State contributes towards maternity benefits.

Sickness funds contract with the associated doctors; and in order that bargaining may be under equal conditions the various sickness funds combine in these negotiations. In these contracts the number of doctors that may be appointed has been limited, only one doctor per 1,000 persons insured being compulsory.[1] This has been the rule since 1923. If the sickness fund and the medical association cannot come to terms, an appeal can be made to the judicial bodies named on page 159.

Dr. Pryll pointed out to me the current difficulties between doctors and sickness funds, and those arising out of the relation of sickness to invalidity insurance. He was of the opinion that private medical practice was dying, and that the conflict of interest between doctors and the public was inevitable.

In Berlin the sickness fund doctor is paid a fixed sum a year for every insured person on his list. In 1926 the payment was 10 to 11 marks, in 1927 it was 12 marks, and in 1928 it had been increased to 13 to 14 marks *per capita*. The details are arranged between the Union of Sickness Funds and the Economic Medical Association. Every insured person going to the doctor of his choice brings with him a card showing that he is insured and entitled to treatment. This ticket is his *bon*. It is retained by the doctor for three months, when the *bons* are counted. The doctor, in addition, makes a return to the Economic Medical Association of the number of visits and consultations, with a separate statement of operations, hypodermic injections, etc. Each of these items has a value of from 2 to 60 points. The aggregate points are compared with

---

[1] In England it is the number of patients per doctor that is limited.

the *bons*. The value of each *bon* decreases as the number of *bons* increases.

The system roughly described above does not conduce to efficient treatment. It is to the doctor's interest to increase the number of *bons*, instead of to give the best treatment possible, and by this means to reduce the duration of medical attendance.[1]

The present system, however, is deeply rooted, and once the contract is made with the Medical Association the sickness fund is not further interested. An enormous staff is engaged in the calculation and correction of the medical accounts, many with high salaries and fees. Thus vested interests have grown up on the medical side which are unfavourable to a simpler and less bureaucratic method of computing medical fees.

The Berlin system appears to preponderate throughout Germany. It is not satisfactory to the doctors themselves, and I doubt if it is in the interest of the insured.

The cost of medical, including dental work, has greatly increased, as may be seen from the following table (Goldmann and Grotjahn, *op. cit.*, p. 23):—

Year	Marks expended on Medical Aid per Member of Sickness Funds	Proportion per cent. of Expenditure on Medical Aid to Total Expenditure
1885	2·11	17·4
1895	3·08	20·4
1905	4·75	20·9
1914	7·47	23·2
1924	14·36	28·7

Note that no separate statement is available giving the proportion of the cost given in the first column which has

[1] *Note dated September* 1930. A recent Presidential Order has been issued, which only allows an insured person to consult a doctor after paying 50 pf. (about 12 cents) for a voucher for this purpose. He must also pay the same sum for every prescription at a pharmacy. Sick funds are also authorised to give a higher money benefit, leaving the insured to make his own medical arrangements. This edict remains valid until confirmed or rejected by the new Reichstag just elected.

been due to introduction of family benefits in the more recent years.

Pathological Aids to Diagnosis are paid for by the sickness funds, and in some large cities these funds have set up diagnostic institutes of their own. There is a large institution for this purpose in Berlin, most of the sickness fund doctors utilising it.

X-ray examinations are also provided for by these funds.

There are special institutes at which electro-physical treatment and treatment by artificial sunlight are given. Some sick funds also possess hydro-therapeutical institutions.

Dental Benefit comes within the scope of sickness insurance, and the replacement of lost teeth within the scope of invalidity insurance, if the general health of the insured is endangered. The extent to which dental diseases are treated varies greatly. In 1925 the annual expenditure for this purpose of all legal sickness funds averaged 2·35 marks per member.

Of the 8,000 dentists in Germany, about 6,000 are said to be employed by the sickness funds.

Drugs.—Similarly, more than half of the work of pharmacists in Germany is for the sickness funds. Insured persons are required to bear 10 per cent. of the cost of drugs and minor appliances; their dependents for the most part a still larger proportion.

Institutional Treatment.—This has been much increased by the desire of the sickness funds to restore working capacity as rapidly as possible, and it is largely owing to this fact that hospitals have ceased to be a provision for the very poor and have become available for everybody. Family dependents are not so well provided for as the insured, though according to the *Sickness Year Book*, 1926, quoted by Goldmann and Grotjahn, 211 funds with nearly 2 million members granted full hospital treatment to dependents, while 620 funds with over 6 million members granted partial hospital treatment.

Some sickness funds possess hospitals of their own, but

usually public hospitals are utilised. Three-fifths of the patients in Berlin municipal hospitals are sent by sickness funds. In large towns it appears that the number of insured receiving hospital treatment when ill varies from one in five to one in thirteen.

There is much discussion as to the inadequacy of the payments made by sick funds for maintenance and treatment of insured sick in municipal hospitals. These are often much below the actual cost. Unlike in England, there is no free treatment of cases of infectious disease in the insured, a considerable additional charge being made for such cases in children who are dependents of the insured. Much institutional treatment is needed in connection with welfare work, whether for insured or non-insured; and it is unfortunate that it should be hampered by the limitations of insurance funds, and not completely forthcoming on public health grounds when patients are unable to pay. It would be well if sickness funds could be prevented from starting and maintaining hospitals of their own. Unified management of hospitals is indispensable to secure the best results.

There is, furthermore, risk of excessive hospitalisation in insurance work. Much of the work now done in hospitals, and especially during convalescence, could be continued at home were medical arrangements, including nursing, available more freely in the home. But this remark has wide application in many countries.

Recently arrangements have been made for treatment at home by city or charitable sisters under medical supervision before and after admission to a hospital. There are also welfare institutions for psychopathics, alcoholics, drug addicts, and cripples.

INVALIDITY INSURANCE

The incidence of invalidity insurance is almost the same as that of insurance against sickness. The contributions of employers and employees are in equal proportions, and there are additional State subsidies. The benefits include invalidity and survivors' pensions, of which we need not give particulars.

The Federal Insurance Code authorised the use of both sickness and invalidity insurance funds for prevention of disease in individual cases, or in the interest of public health; and particulars of such use of these funds are given on pages 147 and 150. It is in regard to tuberculosis that combined curative and preventive work has been most extensively developed. Some particulars of this are given on page 152.

Criticisms of German Sickness and Invalidity Insurance

In the preceding pages some of the embarrassing complexities and difficulties of German insurance have been indicated, and the dissatisfaction of the medical profession with the present position has been stated.

It is difficult to give dispassionately the views of the German physicians whom I interviewed in visits in German centres; but in the following pages some of these are indicated. Fortunately, along with personal impressions, one can utilise a work by Dr. E. Liek, of Dantzig, which probably says the worst that can be advanced against the German system. This work is entitled *Die Schaden der sozialen Versicherung und Wege zur Besserung* (1928, Munchen, J. F. Schmann Verlag). A French translation, *Les Méfaits des Assurances Sociales en Allemagne* (1929, Paris, Payot), with a preface by Professor Georges Weiss, of the Strasburg Faculty of Medicine, is also available.

In this work Dr. Liek, who was for two years a sick fund doctor—but "never again"—states his reasons for thinking the German social insurance in its present form very inimical to the health of the people. This thesis is of vital interest both to practising physicians and to all social workers, and I do not hesitate to summarise his statements in some detail, making comments here and there. The difficulties here summarised are of the very essence of the problem under investigation by me.

When the first stone of the German social insurance edifice was laid in 1883, no consultation with the organised German medical profession was made. This was true in other countries. It was true in England until a late stage of the Bill for sickness insurance was reached, when some unfortunate features could not be remedied. Dr. Liek is confident that in the forty years since 1883 a grave decadence of the medical profession in Germany has been experienced. Some of this admittedly may have been due to the fact that the agricultural population is now only one-third, whereas then it was two-thirds, of the entire population; and that thus relations of personal care have been displaced by legal provisions having more regard for the malady than for the patient.

In considering this problem we must remember the axiom of civilisation that in sickness, poverty, and old age those without means must be cared for by a civilised State. To deny this, to attempt to minimise this responsibility, is to look back towards barbarism.

Long before Bismarck introduced compulsory sickness insurance (1883), the partial ineffectiveness of voluntary attempts had been demonstrated; among others, by Krupp in his factories, who began sickness insurance of his workers on voluntary lines, but was quickly obliged to make it obligatory on all.

At present there are some 70,000 secretaries of workers' sick funds in Germany. In Dr. Liek's opinion, they are the masters of Germany's destiny, in its internal and external relationships. At the beginning, Bismarck's social legislation was carried in opposition to the Social Democrats; now doctors fret and doubt, but workers will not be likely to listen to any attempt to abolish or seriously change this legislation.

From the very beginning there has been intermittent and irritating warfare between practising physicians and the bureaus for whose members they work. There is no doubt that sickness insurance has greatly benefited the insured. The more systematic treatment now given has enabled the masses of the people to benefit from the immense advances made by medical science. Doctors are more promptly consulted; diagnosis is made earlier; and hospital and other services are made available. For the young doctor also the sickness funds have made entry into medical practice easier than in the past. The following are the more serious objections alleged against the present system :—

1. There is the objection, now being urged especially by the French medical profession, that a third party obtrudes into the confidential relationship between doctor and patient.

2. Sickness insurance undermines manliness, encourages effeminacy, and leads to cultivation of ailments.

It is stated by experienced German doctors that two-thirds of the applications for treatment are unnecessary. In the neighbouring country of Poland the sickness funds have a special column in their statistics for "Nihilitis".

The desire and the need to get well expedites recovery to a remarkable extent. This truth has, however, a sinister side, for this desire and need may also lead to incautious and even dangerous return to work.

Dr. Liek is strongly of opinion that the free choice of doctors—a main point in the contention of associated doctors—tends to relaxation of morals; and quotes in this connection statistics showing the large percentages of patients who, on revision of their certification, were found fit for work.

It is notorious that industrial strikes help to fill the consulting-rooms of sick-insurance doctors. Thus often sickness insurance becomes a refuge in economic difficulties more than a means of medical care.

The establishment of unemployment insurance has done much to obviate this abuse, often substituting another in its place.

It may be agreed that if insurance doctors had only sick persons to treat, and if these were all imbued with the wish to recover quickly, much more good could be achieved by the working of sickness insurance.

There are, in fact, many *parasites of insurance*, and these, as Dr. Liek points out, are helped and maintained in their parasitism by a portion of the sickness fund physicians. On the other hand, we may ask, how much suffering would be caused by more rigid restriction of sickness benefits? The ideal can only be reached by a combination of intelligence, judgment, and character on the part of doctors, and of conscientiousness on the part of every person insured, which may be pursued but cannot be completely attained for long years to come.

3. It is contended that the really sick person does not get his deserts.

The inadequate remuneration of the doctor compels him to resort to mass treatment to earn a livelihood for himself and his family. As many as fifty, or even up to 200, may be seen by the doctor in a day's consulting hours; and it is thus exceptional for a person with chest symptoms to be stripped for examination.

Dr. Liek quotes the largest sickness fund of Dantzig, with some 50,000 members, which pays the doctor 6 gulden[1] for each patient treated during three months. From this nominal honorarium nearly a third has to be deducted for general expenses.

In 1925 every German sickness fund doctor received on an average 1·10 marks for a month's treatment, less a deduction of 30 per cent. for expenses. This is compared with the cost of haircutting with a shampoo in Dantzig, which is 1·30 marks! It is true that the sums owing by the sickness funds are actually paid, and that the doctor has a monopoly of treatment, and that through the funds he earns on an average some 9,000 marks per annum, subject to the deduction of one-third indicated above.

4. The administration of the sick funds is very costly. These funds have some 27,000 official employees for the 29,000 doctors engaged in the work, in round numbers. The splendid and luxurious buildings which are to be seen in every large town are symbolical of the immense clerical

[1] 7,000 gulden = 5,775 marks.

organisation of insurance. How many hospitals could have been built with this money! The doctor is "snowed under" by the papers to be signed and returns to be made. In some middle-class funds the management swallows up half the subscriptions. In the compulsory funds of the Empire, management costs 6 per cent. of the total funds.

Dr. Liek instances the case of accidents as showing the extravagance of free choice of doctor. For possibly 100 accidents a day as many doctors may be consulted; whereas at an ambulatorium—available sometimes—there is immensely increased efficiency in treatment and economy in appliances. It surely should be possible to arrange for this in every community.

5. It is commonly stated that sickness insurance has been a great factor in the improved health of Germany. The fact that a majority of the population have medical treatment always available, including admission to hospital when needed, must have been very beneficial. The factors concerned in improved health are, however, complex, as, for instance, in tuberculosis, concerning which Professor Drigalski speaks of the "complete breakdown of the fight" against this disease during the war. In this breakdown collateral influences were operating, including excessive concentrated infection, terrible overcrowding, impoverishment, with deficient clothing and food, etc. One needs to be cautious in assessing the relative importance of various factors which may have influenced the total death-rate.

6. Not only bodily effeminacy but moral deterioration is determined by sickness insurance. Dr. Liek illustrates this by the neurasthenic who, when he consults a new doctor, begs him not to return the same certificate as had previously been given. If he does, there is a further change of doctor. This is a crude illustration of a problem oft-times facing the conscientious doctor.

The above are the general considerations urged by Dr. Liek. He passes on next to the specific drawbacks of insurance work for the doctor from Dr. Liek's viewpoint.

(a) The younger doctor is tempted to multiply his cer-

tificates of unfitness for work, or to magnify minor ailments
—in short, to act as a tradesman, not as a physician.

(*b*) Treatment *en masse* means careless clinical work. For
this the overwhelming clerical work is partly to blame.

Free choice of doctor conduces rather to lightning
diagnosis than to accurate work. Although the income
earned by insurance doctors is small, that is not the most
regrettable feature of their insurance work. It is rather that
the earning of this money too often implies hasty work,
cultivation of ailments, and unnecessary treatment. If a
doctor takes up the necessary time for a serious case,
others with trifling ailments go elsewhere. This argument
appears to me to overreach the mark. It might apply to
any popular doctor in large practice outside sickness
insurance. Doubtless, however, something is lost in the
patient not being obliged to assess the value of his consultation with the doctor by direct payment.

(*c*) The intimate relation between doctor and patient is
rendered more difficult in insurance work. For private
patients the doctor is concerned only with the patient's
illness; in insurance work he has to consider also whether
the patient is only wanting a certificate. The doctor is then
a detective for the sickness fund. But he is also dependent
for his livelihood on the good will of the insured person
consulting him.

(*d*) Massive work leaves no time for study or recreation.
Apart from the excessive clinical work, there is the "eternal
writing", most of it unnecessary.

(*e*) The facility with which the medical beginner can
make a practice tempts many not fit for it to study medicine.
But there is no calling in which so little is earned for so
much hard work.

The sickness funds themselves say there are too many
doctors; and on this they are able to base the low payments
given for medical work. There follows the superficial treatment of symptoms, and so the vicious circle is complete.

(*f*) Sickness fund practice has democratised the practice
of medicine. This may, however, be regarded as a com-

mendation of sickness insurance. Treatment is more generally available than ever in the past. But it has been followed
by extensions of insurance, wider and wider social circles
demanding a cheapened medical service. Collective contracts
made by the Leipzig Federation have minimised this evil;
but still more and more doctors and more and more
patients are brought under the yoke of contract practice.

Invalidity insurance comes even more under the lash of
Dr. Liek's pen. It has an immense administrative machinery,
a gigantic organisation, the chief benefit from which in
Germany is the payment of 35 marks a month to the
invalid—"too little to live and too much to die". This
statement leaves out of account the valuable care organisations associated with invalidity insurance, and especially for
tuberculosis.

Dr. Liek's objections to social insurance extend to social
welfare work carried out by voluntary bodies and public
health authorities. In his opinion, this welfare work fosters
illness more than care of health! Insurance schemes are
regarded as special evidence of advanced civilisation, but
to Dr. Liek it seems possible that they may lead to the
downfall of civilisation. The consulting-room, in his view,
is no more a temple in which the sick man seeks healing,
but an exchange in which business is transacted.

The damage done to the soul by unworthily seeking for
insurance benefits cannot be restored by money.

In summing up, Dr. Liek concludes that insurance, while
useful to the individual, is highly mischievous to the people
as a whole.

I must not be taken as agreeing with this or other statements of Dr. Liek; but a summary of his work gives a
useful recapitulation of whatever can be said against social
insurance as practised in Germany.

Much less can one agree with the Swiss doctor (quoted
by Dr. Liek without agreement) who maintains that
Germany "lost the war because her nervous system had
been damaged by social insurances".

It will be convenient, as giving a useful focus of the

problems concerned, to follow Dr. Liek further in his discussion of the remedies for the alleged mischief caused by German social insurance.

The first remedy is the removal of the "cultivation of sickness". With this abstract proposition there will be general agreement. Dr. Liek contends that better payment of doctors would not remedy the present evil. There are, in his view, only two possible ways: either the repeal of social insurance, or its complete reorganisation. The first of these is obviously impracticable. A large majority of the German population lives from hand to mouth, and would be helpless without social insurance.

It is generally agreed that the insured are of two classes: those who want to get well, and those who don't. The latter try to make a business of being ill. Hence the struggle of the sick funds to convert the doctors into officials, while the doctors, on their part, insist on the insured having free choice of doctors.

Very few doctors are outside the two great medical organisations, the Aerzte Vereinsbund and Hartmann Bund, and these enable the medical profession to secure some amelioration of the conditions of medical service, though politically they cannot compete against the millions of organised working men and women.

Extensions of social insurance intensify the problem. There are now sickness funds for the middle classes and for officials. There is a project for compulsory sickness insurance for the highest officials. This Poland has had for some years.

The medical profession is overcrowded. Many young doctors are unemployed; often there is prolonged waiting before a vacancy occurs in a sick fund.

The figures of German income-tax are significant of the narrow margin still available for private medical practice. According to Hadrich (*Aertzliche Mittheilungen*, 1927), there are about four million people liable to pay income-tax. Of these four millions, 75 per cent. have an income not exceeding 5,000 marks per annum.

Evidently, with an upper limit of 6,000 marks for social insurance, private practice has small scope. Dr. Liek' remedy is drastic. There are three conceivable possibilities:—

(1) A reorganisation of the medical profession, with national unification of the insurance service, along with a complete free choice of doctors. This, however, would merely intensify existing bureaucracy.

(2) In considering English methods, he concludes that, to a mitigated extent, there are the same difficulties in England as in Germany.

(3) He pleads in favour of making the sickness fund doctor a State official. While disliking this, Dr. Liek considers this the less of two evils, and as giving to the free doctors their last chance of salvation.

In his opinion this complete officialisation (if this word is permissible) of the sickness fund doctor would make it possible for him to become also a medical officer of health in the region of his medical work. At present, with the system of *bons*, a healthy period means an empty consulting-room and anxiety for wife and family. With a complete official salary this anxiety would disappear, and the doctor could become the health adviser of the family. The present competition for patients would cease, and the doctor would not be subject to the temptation to favour the patient unfairly at the expense of the sick fund. When epidemics occurred, it would then be practicable to draft doctors where they were specially needed.

Of course, under such a scheme the doctor's freedom would be gone; but Dr. Liek urges that it has already disappeared; and a State official has greater freedom than a sickness fund official. Bureaucracy would not be reduced, nor would it be increased.

At present a quarter of the physicians in Germany give some of their time to social medical work for the State or local authorities in Fürsorge (welfare) stations. Hospital doctors do not neglect their patients because of inadequate salaries.

It is true that an official doctor will then replace the doctor in whom the patient has personal confidence. But the choice of doctors even now is based most often on most casual considerations, and at ambulatoria and in hospitals it does not exist.

Hospitals already, in Dr. Liek's view, have broken the back of private practice; and in Germany they have very commonly "undercut" expert private practice, as well as the private clinics for paying patients, which find it difficult to continue.

I do not propose to follow Dr. Liek's arguments further at this stage; they are placed on record, and will be weighed in a separate volume, when I discuss the merits and demerits of sickness insurance in different European countries.

THE STATE OF HAMBURG [1]

Among Germany's seventeen constituent States, special historic interest attaches to the three Free Hanseatic States of Bremen, Hamburg, and Lubeck, with their long-time experience of almost completely autonomous government. But they form constituent States of the German Empire, and as such bear their share of Imperial taxation, and have the same service of social insurance as the rest of Germany. The control of the Imperial Government over the local expenditure of money derived from Imperial taxation is relatively small.

Hamburg is governed by a House of Burgesses (Bürgerschaft) of 160 members. These elect an executive Senate of sixteen members, its chief member being the Burgomaster, who possesses more executive power than an English mayor. The State consists of the city of Hamburg, with a population in 1930 of 1,143,079, and a surrounding area containing 83,032 people.

Public health authority is vested in a Board of Health,

[1] Date of this inquiry, June 1930. A good account of public health organisation in Hamburg is given by Surgeon J. G. Townsend, of the U.S. Public Health Service, in *Public Health Reports*, November 22, 1929,

elected by the Bürgerschaft. It comprises two senators, eight citizens, and one financial member. The members of this board hold office for four years, two retiring each year, but they may be re-elected. This arrangement implies delegation of executive power to a body not directly elected by the people, subject only to financial control by the Bürgerschaft. Two officers are attached to this board, one medical, one non-medical, who have security of tenure of office, retiring at the age of sixty-five, in accordance with the general official rule.

Under the Board of Health are two whole-time medical officers of health for the city of Hamburg, to one of whom, Dr. G. Herman Sieveking, I am indebted for valuable help. This joint arrangement for the city is said to work smoothly. There are separate officers for Cuxhaven and Bergersdorf in the State of Hamburg.

In the city of Hamburg there are fourteen district or community medical officers, who attend the sick poor, are called in for accidents, and do general police medical work.

In Altona (Prussia) the community doctor is also medical officer of health; and this combination, the "community doctor" doing dispensary work for the poor as well as public health work, holds good in some larger cities in Prussia. Where the "community doctor" is independent of the medical officer of health there is some reduction of efficiency and liability to friction.

Some of the private practitioners are employed as public vaccinators, being paid per hour for this work. No payment is made to practitioners for medical notifications of cases of infectious sickness. The two medical officers of health can call on the fourteen medical officers for help when required.

Vaccination is controlled by a special organisation at the Vaccine Institute, and is enforced by the police. It is compulsory in the first calendar year after the year of birth and again in the twelfth year. All school-children must show satisfactory evidence of vaccination before admission to school. A small fee is charged to doctors for vaccine lymph for their own patients.

There are also five whole-time "Court" physicians, whose duties are forensic in character, and who arrange for the treatment of the insane, undertake autopsies, etc. They also determine the medical fitness of teachers and other officials.

Pathological material from infectious diseases is examined free for practitioners at the Hygienic Institute.

SOCIAL WELFARE ORGANISATIONS

While there are fourteen city districts with provision for sick care of the poor by fourteen part-time doctors appointed by the Board of Health, the city is divided into eleven (not fourteen) areas in which the work of three central boards is carried on. These are :—

1. The Board of Health under which works the Hamburg Public Health Service (Gesundheitsbehorde).
2. The Board of Public Welfare for the Poor (Wohlfahrtsbehorde). This does the work of what has been known hitherto in England as poor law relief.
3. The Board for the Young (Jugendbehorde).

These three boards receive independent appropriations from the Government. Together they are known as Gesundheits-Fürsorge or Welfare Organisation; and the efficiency of their collective work depends on the measure of co-operation and intercommunication between them.

In each of the eleven districts of the city is one or more welfare centres, which serve for general welfare work, for infant consultations, and as tuberculosis dispensaries.

Nurses from the first of these boards make visits at homes where infectious cases have been notified, largely at the request of the district doctors. The nurses of the second board work in collaboration with them, and deal largely with the social problems of the poor, such as care of infancy and admission to hospital beds; while the nurses of the third board are concerned with the welfare of illegitimate children and foster-children boarded out in private homes. They also collaborate in visiting the mothers of all infants who are entitled to insurance benefits while actually nursing their infants.

There are also four chief voluntary welfare societies engaged in similar work:—

1. The Society for Improving the Health of the People (Landesverband für Volksgesundheitspflege).
2. The Committee for Institutional Care of Children (Ausschuss für Kinderanstalten).
3. The Association for Care of Cripples (Verein für Krüppelfürsorge).
4. The Central Organisation for the Care of Infants and Young Children (Landeszentrale für Sanglings und Kleinkinder-Schutz).

These bodies have now become in large measure quasi-official, as voluntary contributions are small.

We may now consider the combined work of these organisations as affecting maternity and child welfare and efforts against tuberculosis.

There are no municipal *midwives*, but the municipality pays for attendance on the very poor in childbirth. It also pays for maternity beds in the lying-in hospitals. In these hospitals patients can secure accommodation in three classes, according to the degree of privacy. Occasionally insurance societies pay for a consultant doctor when needed by a midwife. Three-fourths of the total births in the city occur in hospitals. Special antenatal work has only recently been begun. Public health nurses (belonging to No. 4 above) do not visit the homes until eight days after a birth has occurred; before this the doctor or midwife is responsible. The insurance societies give a benefit of 1 mark a week for six weeks after confinement for the wives of insured persons, and home visits are made incidentally to serve the purpose of inspection in this as well as in other respects. The insurance society pays the municipality for the work done by the public health nurse in supervising breast-feeding. If patients are very poor and there is no insurance benefit, the welfare centre may pay the same amount for thirteen weeks. A weekly sum is also paid by insurance societies for six weeks before the confinement; and 40 marks are paid to the midwife if the patient is confined at home. Most cases, however, go to the hospital, sickness insurance funds paying for this provision.

The number of health visitors or public health nurses dealing with child welfare was only ten in 1914; in 1930 there were 112. Each of these is stated to make about 300 home visits in a month.

The *Infant Consultations* are conducted by part-time physicians, who are paid 10 marks for each attendance of one to two hours.

They see all the children brought to the centre. There are altogether thirty-two of these centres, at which children up to the age of six are seen. The bringing of older children is stimulated by giving food cards to the poor; and that of mothers with infants is fairly general, as the payment to the nursing mother of a mark a week depends on the doctor's or nurse's certificate. It is estimated that not less than 95 per cent. of infants born are seen by the nurses, most of them several times.

There has been some friction with private doctors, although the welfare doctors refrain from treating the sick. This has arisen from the legitimate objection that the part-time doctor conducting the centre obtains a "pull" in securing private patients by this work. To obviate this objection, it has been decided that no doctor shall work at the centre which is in the district of his private practice, which should obviate the reasonable jealousies of private practitioners.

At *Tuberculosis Dispensaries* no treatment is carried out. At first part-time doctors were employed, and paid per hour. Now whole-time specialist tuberculosis physicians are employed. There has been some agitation against these dispensaries, in view of the fear that patients would be treated. The visiting nurses have specialised in this work. They meet daily and exchange notes with the infant and welfare workers. The Reich has now made regulations insisting on two years' training of public health nurses and a compulsory examination.

It should be added that both child welfare and tuberculosis nurses visit private doctors and offer their services for cases in private medical practice.

The visits to tuberculosis patients at home are made monthly. There is no compulsory notification of cases, but they become known through the insurance offices and by attendance at the dispensaries. They are sent to the dispensaries by insurance doctors and from hospitals, or may come independently. It is stated that 15 per cent. of all the cases are sent by private doctors for diagnosis.

There are altogether six tuberculosis districts, each with a special physician for tuberculosis. Each of these physicians has four district nurses attached to four sub-districts. One Röntgen-ray outfit is supplied for four of the districts.

The tuberculosis nurses are authorised by the municipality to pay each inadequately housed family the sum of 40 marks monthly to supplement the provision of houseroom. The Invalidity Insurance Society pays one-half of these grants. This has been in operation (June 1930) for six months, and will be continued as long as the funds are available. This work imposes a heavy administrative burden on the nurses, but it gives them great influence in enforcing a hygienic life.

There are adequate institutional beds for the treatment of tuberculosis. At present there is no compulsory power to remove patients, but such an enactment is contemplated.

VENEREAL DISEASES

There are no special clinics for these diseases, except those attached to general hospitals. For the treatment of most cases the insurance societies are responsible, paying hospitals for treatment according to a scale. In this, and in other diseases, the municipality regard the payments made by insurance societies as inadequate.

SCHOOL MEDICAL WORK

This work is under the Board of Health, medical inspections being made by part-time doctors, under a part-time chief school medical officer. Each school doctor has the schools in a single district allotted to him. No treatment is carried out in connection with school medical inspection, this being rendered almost unnecessary because most children are entitled to medical care under the sickness insurance organisation. The sickness societies, for instance, have skilled ophthalmic surgeons, and they pay for the hospital treatment of adenoids, etc. Thorough dental treatment is undertaken by the school medical service, the children usually paying a small fee.

The school medical service in the above circumstances naturally arouses no opposition from private medical practitioners.

Hospitals

There are three public hospitals, two hospitals for the insane, and three special hospitals in Hamburg City, having altogether 12,400 beds. The entire staff of these hospitals are in the Government service and under the general supervision of the Board of Health. At private hospitals there are 3,560 additional beds.

All patients treated in hospitals are paid for.

(1) The majority of sick persons in the community receive treatment as part of their sick benefit, the insurance societies paying the Board of Health for this in accordance with a specified scale. This payment only suffices to cover part of the expense of hospital treatment. Sickness insurance is thus largely subsidised out of general taxation.

(2) All persons not coming within the first class above (that is, those with wages up to 3,600 marks, or 850 dollars a year), but with a salary between this amount and 8,400 marks a year, are also insured; and they thereby ensure hospital provision when ill. Thus is solved the problem of hospital provision for the lower middle and middle classes, who in Great Britain and some other countries find themselves in serious difficulty when needing hospital treatment. In many towns in Britain a voluntary hospital contributing scheme is helping to fill this gap.

(3) The same hospitals provide treatment for the well-to-do. These can secure private rooms in the hospital by appropriate payment.

(4) This leaves a small group of non-insured persons who are destitute, for whom the municipality is responsible.

There appears to be no complaint on the part of private doctors of excessive hospitalisation of cases of illness. The sickness insurance system renders this unlikely.

SICKNESS INSURANCE

Sickness insurance is compulsory in Hamburg under Federal law (see p. 158). For sickness insurance the worker pays two-thirds and the employer one-third of the weekly contribution; for old age and invalidity insurance, each of these pays one-half. The premiums for accident insurance are paid by the employer only. The premiums for sickness and invalidity insurance vary, as also the monetary benefit, according to the wages of the insured. The insured person's wife and children receive medical benefit, and this includes consultation services and hospital provision. Doctors are paid for their individual work for insured persons by "points" according to the work done (see also p. 167).

Each consultation at the doctor's surgery counts as one "point".

A visit to the patient's home counts as three "points".

Special fees attach to more detailed examination and operations.

About five-eighths of the physicians in Hamburg are engaged in insurance work. The number is kept restricted to one doctor per 1,000 persons insured. Younger doctors have difficulty in obtaining this work, often having to wait three or four years before they can come on the list, and meanwhile they find it difficult to live. In the whole of Germany there are stated to be 3,000 doctors thus waiting to be employed.

The monetary arrangements between the organised doctors and the three chief insurance societies of Hamburg are made without any intermediary (in England the Central Government acts in this capacity). The insurance societies make their own arrangements with the municipality for hospital treatment of the insured. The insurance organisation has four large buildings in which medical referees sit to decide on cases of difficulty, including supposed malingering. At these centres are also special polyclinics for the insured; and an insurance doctor can always obtain expert advice for a patient at these. Insured persons are only admitted to a polyclinic on the recommendation of a doctor. The affairs of each insurance society are controlled by a committee which gives equal representation to employers and to workers; the general arrangements are controlled at the local general Sick Insurance Institute, which acts also as a consultative and referee centre. This referee organisation is very complete and business-like; and the doctors in charge of it, although employed by the insurance societies, appeared to me to hold the balance skilfully between these insurance societies and the insurance doctors. The insured person when sick takes a card to the doctor of his choice, on one portion of which the latter writes his diagnosis, this constituting his claim for payment. Every such card comes to the referee office, and the office pays 7 marks per case, with additional "points" according to the number of visits made or other special work. Each doctor's work is analysed at the office. The average cost per patient for all doctors is known, and the particular doctor is marked off periodically as having had the average experience or x per cent. more or less than this. The doctor with unusual experience is interviewed by the referee doctor, if excessive cost continues to coincide with his work. This is said to work wholesomely without much friction. It is not regarded as tending to inadequate medical attendance. I gathered the impression that this view in the main was correct.

The insurance doctors are appointed by the insurance societies with the limitation already indicated. In practice each patient has the choice of two or three doctors in his own district. These doctors also engage in such private practice as they can secure. As the wives and children of the insured come within the range of insurance practice, the scope for private practice is correspondingly limited. At the present time there is agitation among Hamburg practitioners, especially the younger, to secure the patient's absolutely free choice of doctor. This is already given in Munich and some other areas. Each doctor in Hamburg can send his patient to a specialist at one of the four large polyclinics for this purpose when he thinks this desirable. Patients can change their doctors, but not easily.

In Greater Hamburg there are about 540,000 insured persons, for whom, according to the limit stated above, there should be 540 doctors. In fact, 635 doctors are engaged in the work of sickness insurance.

Interviewing a distinguished consultant in Hamburg, I was informed that sickness insurance has greatly decreased the clientele of all private practitioners, including that of consultant physicians. In particular the societies' medical plan of *numerus clausus* has caused much medical privation since the war. The abstraction from private practice through insurance work has shown itself markedly in the difficulty which private hospitals and nursing-homes now experience to secure patients. The public hospitals of the municipality receive insured patients at the rate of 6·80 marks, while 12 marks are required to pay expenses. There are still some hospitals (Protestant, Red Cross, Jewish, Methodist, Free-masons, and Catholic) supported from private funds; but 90 per cent. of all hospital patients are treated in the municipal hospitals. The handicap of private institutions is increased by the fact that these, unlike charitable and municipal hospitals, have to pay taxes and receive no subsidy from the State.

From the above short summary it is evident that the position between doctors and insurance societies is much less strained in Hamburg than in Berlin.

Even as to the complaint of young doctors that they cannot secure work, it may be contended that they merely share the difficulties experienced by lawyers and other professional workers.

I had the advantage of discussing the entire subject with Professor Dr. Albrecht Mendelssohn-Bartolomy, Professor of the Department of Politics in the University of Hamburg, and with Dr. Madalena Schoch, Assistant Professor of Social Economics, and from them and from other sources I was given the social view and the view of the insured, which is even more important than that of the insurance doctors, although without the active and sympathetic co-operation of the last named sickness insurance cannot be completely successful. It is well to remember, however :—

(1) That social, including sickness insurance, in Germany is so popular that a large proportion of the population who are outside its compulsory scope join voluntarily the sickness and invalidity insurance societies, or special voluntary societies. In the last named the insured person pays his own private doctor, and the bill is then sent to the insurance society, which pays it entirely—if the doctor is willing to accept the scale of fees adopted by the society—or part of it in other cases. Evidently the doctor runs some risk of not being paid in this arrangement. In these voluntary societies there is no contribution by employers. The State may be said to contribute indirectly by its general super-vision of the financial position of each society. Many municipal and State officials join such societies, and the tendency in professional and skilled occupations to do likewise appears to be increasing.

(2) There can be no reasonable doubt that in the present circumstances of Germany a large part of the population, in the absence of insurance, would suffer from more or less medical neglect. This occurred to some extent before sickness insurance existed, when there was less poverty and unemployment than now.

There has been great improvement not only in the almost complete cessation of lack of medical care, and the substitution for it of assured domiciliary medical care and of specialist aid and of hospital treatment, but also in the fact that a buttress has been built against destitution by the weekly financial allowances provided by insurance. These two forms of aid have a high social value, the importance of which can scarcely be exaggerated.

(3) Although many German doctors are dissatisfied with the present conditions of insurance medical work, and there is indeed need for improvements, the balance of evidence points to the conclusion that the remedy lies in part with the doctors themselves, in their individual and collective capacity.

I should add that the doctor's position in one important particular is more conducive to good work under the British plan than in Germany, in that the financial conditions of work of insurance doctors are decided by negotiation between the Government and the organised doctors. The adoption of such a procedure in Germany would greatly help to reduce present medical dissatisfaction. But the scope of medical treatment in the German is more nearly complete, and therefore more satisfactory, than in the English system. It would be possible in Germany, as elsewhere, to pay doctors more generously were due care exercised by them all without exception to give their attendance on patients strictly in accordance with medical needs and regardless of other considerations, and to certify illness without bias in favour of the patient. The duties of doctors necessitate tact and judgment and a meticulous sense of honour, and the obstacles to their fulfilment are obvious. They can be overcome when all doctors have fully realised the implications of their work, and when they support each other in doing what sometimes is necessarily unpopular in regard to individual patients. This does not imply that they become primarily the agents of the insurance society, and that they consider insurance finance rather than the patient's welfare; but it does mean a balanced judgment and a conscientious execution of work in the spirit of equity. This spirit doubtless actuates the majority of doctors, but, as in other countries, a minority render inevitable the making of exact and precise regulations and checks on medical action; and these regulations and checks are necessarily irksome and irritating, and especially to those for whom they are not needed.

The need to limit medical attendance to what is really needed in the patient's interest raises the important question whether this may not imply that early recourse to medical aid, which may shorten illness and have definite preventive value, is impeded and restricted. This point will be more adequately discussed in a separate volume. It is only necessary to state at this point that the experience gathered in Germany and elsewhere has convinced me (a) that persons really needing medical attendance are seldom prevented, when medical advice is their right, from seeking it whenever needed; and (b) that in present circumstances undue resort to doctors mainly implies a perfunctory interview with the doctor, no attempt at an exact diagnosis, and encouragement of the view that a "bottle of medicine" is the great desideratum, not the medical or hygienic advice which generally should take its place.

(4) As occurs elsewhere, there is in Germany frequent recourse to sickness benefit when an insured person is unemployed (but is not eligible for unemployment benefits) or unemployable. Sometimes, again, insured persons tired of their work will apply to their doctor for a certificate of sick benefit enabling them to get a week's holiday or "Christmas benefit" not at their own expense. These are a few among many illustrations of the intellectual and moral difficulties besetting a doctor in the conscientious discharge of his duty as a medical certifier. They illustrate the further fact that the insured themselves, much more than the doctors, need to have a conscientious regard for the ethics of certification. This point is common to sickness insurance in all countries. It might be partially remedied by organised addresses and appeals to all insured workers.

Insurance is not a savings bank out of which one is entitled to withdraw what one has put in, irrespective of need; but a provision for the distribution of risks and burdens, by payments which thus become minimal, and by which the fortunate help the unfortunate.

If in such addresses appeal is made to the co-operative motive, and if the analogous cases of insurance against fire or against automobile accidents are utilised in illustration, the nature of the contract in sickness insurance should become more generally realised. The same analogy should help to bring home to all insured persons that by adopting a mode of life consistent with the laws of health they can reduce the amount of sickness, and so prepare the way for larger benefits when sickness does occur.

But these considerations are general, and not special to those persons who are insured against sickness in Germany.

CHAPTER VI

AUSTRIA[1]

PRELIMINARY SUMMARY

Austria is struggling with great national difficulties with much success. Notwithstanding these difficulties, it has elaborate medical provision at the expense of the public purse.

Births occur very largely in institutions in cities. Every commune is legally bound to provide a salaried midwife, her income being supplemented by private practice. Puerperal sepsis is excessive. So also is tuberculosis.

There is a very complete system of compulsory social insurance. The method of payment for domiciliary medical attendance under it varies. It is supplemented in elaborate polyclinics, and medical benefit also includes hospital treatment.

The hospital system is maintained by the taxpayer, subject to what can be recovered from patients. Insurance societies pay a part of the charge for insured patients, and other patients who can pay are charged. The deficit comes out of provincial and national funds.

Austria in its after-the-war position presents many problems of great interest to the hygienist and physician. These are largely governed by its economic position, the story of which is fairly well known.

As determined by the Treaty of St. Germain, September 10, 1919, Austria has a territory of 83,770 square kilometres, as compared with its former 300,004 square kilometres, and a population of 6,535,385 (March 1923), as compared with 28,571,934 (December 1910). The Austro-Hungarian Monarchy had been dissolved, one of the Succession States becoming the Republic of Austria; but, notwithstanding many changes, its social fabric and its medico-hygienic arrangements still partake largely of the

[1] Date of investigation, May 1929.

former position, with its associated centralised paternalism and decentralised provincial autonomy.

Economically, Austria is now slowly recovering from its financial calamities, but with conditions and obligations which still tell heavily against possibilities of active hygienic work. The intellectual classes have become almost as poor as the manual workers; and, were it not for the system of pensions for all employees of the State and municipalities, official workers would be in a not much better frame. The collapse of the former currency meant, on the one hand, a wiping out for a few pence of collective debts, and of mortgages on houses, etc.; on the other hand, it destroyed the savings on which many hundreds of thousands depended for maintenance; and this has implied treatment in public hospitals, at the common expense, of multitudes who formerly would have employed and paid their own doctors. Private medical practice has been further restricted by the unwillingness of the so-called middle and upper classes to call in a doctor for anything less than an evident urgent need.

Rent restriction illustrates the evil position. The raising of rents was forbidden in 1922 by a Federal Act, and this law is still maintained. As a result rents on premises occupied before this time and still occupied by the same tenant are extremely low, and one great need of the labouring and other classes who live in these apartments is met at a minimum pre-war cost; but, on the other hand, owners of houses, many of whom are now poorer than the workers, are almost ruined, and workmen who have changed their dwellings are paying exorbitant rents. A workman's apartment may cost only two to three Austrian shillings a month (1·70 shillings = an English shilling, or about 24 cents); whereas in the open market, if the house had been built since 1922, the rent would be many times higher than this. It is true that the tenant is under an obligation to contribute a proportion of the cost of repairs and dilapidations, which varies with the size of the apartment; but this does not mean an equitable distribution of expenditure, or a satisfactory rental on the property. There is, in fact, an evil circle, formed of the low earnings of the people, the unsatisfactory economic position of the State, and the unfair exploitation of the owner of house property, from which the Government apparently dare not break loose by any method which will mean justice for the owner of houses, while restricting his profit within a reasonable limit.[1]

An unskilled worker in Vienna, one, for instance, who is engaged in transport work, will receive 40 to 50 Austrian shillings a week. This is a usual wage in various occupations.

Although rents for dwellings occupied since before the war are almost nominal, there is in Vienna a municipal tax on every occupied room, very heavily graduated upwards, but still for the poorest dwellings a material addition to rents. Every employer must pay a sum varying from 4 to 8 per cent. on the wages and salaries of persons employed by him. Hotels pay 10 per cent. of their receipts. We cannot follow the complex and varied methods of indirect taxation, some of them special to Vienna. Notwithstanding these, it is claimed by the President of the Vienna Diet that the taxation of the people of Vienna is now no higher than in 1913. This remarkable result, if it bears analysis, must be largely due to the pre-war indebtedness of the capital having been repaid during the currency depreciation by a sum which is fantastically small.

Notwithstanding the serious calamities which have befallen Austria, there is evidence of improving social conditions in some respects. The President of the Viennese Diet boasts of its being the only city which is governed by a Socialist Majority. Many social experiments have been begun in a time of financial distress, and this is not the place to pass judgment on them. Public services have been created which most persons outside the Viennese Diet

[1] By a compromise effected during 1929, some improvement will be gradually effected, slow increases being allowed in the rental of middle- and lower-class flats in Vienna. The increases allowed will only bring new rents up to one-fifth of their pre-war value by the end of 1929.

would regard as better left to private enterprise. They
include the running of a brewery. Perhaps there is more to
be said for a municipal Funeral Furnishing Service, with
a view to the diminution of financial stress when family
bereavement occurs. But a more moderate practice is
emerging; and Vienna, as well as the rest of Austria, which
is more conservative than its capital, will probably succeed
in "making good" in its present more limited domain.
Denmark was quoted to me as an example of a small
country to be emulated. Austria is steadily becoming more
self-dependent. It has begun to produce its own sugar.
Now it has milk and butter enough without importation;
and although the importation of wheat continues, a larger
proportion is now being grown in Austria. A chief need
is coal, the lack of which is inadequately compensated by
water power. The yearly national income is now balanced:
and the great need appears to be more capital for development of new industries and agriculture.

Public Administration

In essential particulars public health administration is
identical with that of the former Dual Monarchy. The
Republic has an Assembly (Nationalrat) elected by popular
vote, and a First Chamber (Bundesrat), consisting of forty-
six members and chosen by the provincial assemblies in
proportion to population. There are nine provinces, each
of which has a provincial assembly (Landtag) elected by
the people of the province. This has only one chamber.
Each province has a special board of health and a whole
time medical officer.

Each province is divided into *Political Administrative
Districts* (Bezirkshauptmannschaften), of which there are
ninety-four, excluding Vienna (which ranks as a province);
and these districts are divided into *Communes*, with councils,
the members of which are elected by the people. Each
commune has a burgomaster and a special administrative
committee. The relation of these to one another and to
the Central Government is seen in the following scheme:—

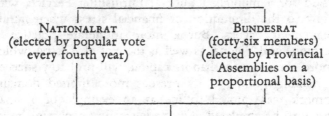

PRESIDENT OF REPUBLIC
(elected by Nationalrat and Bundesrat)

NATIONALRAT
(elected by popular vote
every fourth year)

BUNDESRAT
(forty-six members)
(elected by Provincial
Assemblies on a
proportional basis)

NINE PROVINCIAL COUNCILS
(Assembly [Landtag] elected by popular vote)

NINETY-FOUR POLITICAL ADMINISTRATIVE COUNCILS

COMMUNAL COUNCILS

The Central Government has a *Ministry of Social Administration* (Bundesministerium für Soziale Verwaltung). The *National Public Health Office* (Volksgesundheitsamt) is a special department of this Ministry.

The National Public Health Office is divided into a number of sections, in which are supervised and partially controlled the various local services bearing on insurance, health, hospitals, medical and midwifery practice, control of communicable diseases, vaccination, legislation, etc., in which we are interested.

Poor Law Administration is in charge of the Ministry of the Interior; but in the provinces the same authorities control relief and public health. Factory inspection is in a department of the Ministry of Social Administration, separate from that of Public Health.

PROVINCIAL ADMINISTRATION

Each of the nine provinces of Austria has an appointed physician (Director of the Public Health Department) who does not practise private medicine. He supervises the medical officers in each district in the province. The provincial medical officers are appointed directly by the President of the Austrian Republic—a survival of the centralised

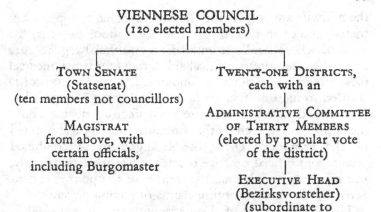

VIENNESE COUNCIL
(120 elected members)

TOWN SENATE
(Statsenat)
(ten members not councillors)

MAGISTRAT
from above, with
certain officials,
including Burgomaster

TWENTY-ONE DISTRICTS,
each with an

ADMINISTRATIVE COMMITTEE
OF THIRTY MEMBERS
(elected by popular vote
of the district)

EXECUTIVE HEAD
(Bezirksvorsteher)
(subordinate to
Burgomaster for Vienna)

control of the former Empire. There are 112 district medical officers. They are now required to have special training. They must, after receiving their medical qualification, have been internes in a hospital for two years, and must then pass a special examination in forensic medicine, hygiene, sanitation, psychology, pharmacy, chemistry, public health law, bacteriology, and the prevention of communicable diseases.

The districts are divided again into communes, each of which is under a legal obligation to provide general medical and midwifery services for the poor.

Communal doctors may be appointed by the communal council, when their salary is paid entirely by the commune. In rural districts where communes are unable to pay the doctor's salary out of local rates the province contributes to the pay-roll of the communal doctor. In these cases the Provincial Diet exercises the right to approve the appointment of the communal doctor. Several smaller communes may join to appoint a communal doctor.

It is a duty of the communes to give both material help and medical assistance for sickness in the poor. The payment for medical attendance is rendered by the commune in the form of an annual salary to the doctor.

The salaries paid to the communal medical officer and to

the midwife are very small. They are expected to supplement their incomes in private practice. Only poor persons, the head of whose family is entered on an official register, are entitled to gratuitous medical aid. Others must pay medical fees, which are minimal in amount. The medical officer is entitled to increase them if he can. In Lower Austria it has been found difficult to secure a satisfactory doctor under the conditions offered by the commune, and he is appointed by the Provincial Diet. The arrangement of combined private and official practice is stated to work satisfactorily, and it is not thought that the welfare of the poor is endangered by the more tempting claims of paying patients.

The attractiveness of these appointments is increased in most provinces by old age pensions to doctors. In Lower Austria the pension is higher than the salary before the pension becomes due, i.e. after thirty-five years of service, or earlier if the doctor is incapacitated, when a partial pension is given.

The district medical officer undertakes vaccination gratuitously for all applicants. This is not compulsory in Austria. The communal medical officer is responsible not only for the treatment of the poor, but also for first-aid in accidents; and he must have a deputy on duty when he is away from home. Public hospitals are required to admit patients sent to them, if found to be suitable for hospital treatment. Poor patients are treated without personal charge, but at the expense of the province to which they belong; others pay according to their means.

The Federal Government contributes yearly a sum of 28·5 million shillings for local public work, which is distributed by the Provincial Diets. The medical officers are placed on a definite scale of increasing salaries. They cannot be dismissed except for misconduct, and each such case must be considered by a jury appointed by the Ministry.

HOSPITAL ADMINISTRATION

Most of the Austrian hospitals are built and maintained at the public expense. The private or voluntary hospitals

are also subject to ministerial supervision with some measure
of control in medical matters. Fortnightly statistical returns
to the Ministry of Social Welfare are demanded from each
hospital, and there are exact statistics of the work being done.

In the public hospitals the charges are fixed by the
governors of the provinces. Krankenkassen must pay
9·70 shillings (Austrian) a day for each insured patient who
is admitted to a public hospital in Vienna in the third class.
In rural hospitals the charge varies between 6 and 7 shillings
a day. As the average cost *per diem* in Vienna is 11 shillings,
a deficit results on the treatment of the insured, as well as
on that of the poorer uninsured patients. This deficit is
made up in the following way :—

1. Two-eighths is paid by the body maintaining the hospital
   (a voluntary organisation or municipality),
2. Three-eighths by the Provincial Government,
3. Three-eighths by the Federal Government.

There is a fairly complete system of hospitals for the entire
country; even in rural districts hospitals are normally
within reach. It is, furthermore, noteworthy that there are
many more medical beds (probably double) than surgical
beds.

The difficulties of housing have increased the impetus to
provide hospital accommodation; and other exigencies of
medical insurance work have increased the pressure in this
direction. It does not appear likely that the desire to "shunt"
insurance patients has influenced the number of hospital
patients : in rural districts the insurance doctor is paid not
on an annual basis, but nearly always per attendance made.
It is believed, however, that there is some "hyper-hospital-
ism", and the hospital beds are often unnecessarily occupied,
as, for instance, for incurable diseases. But if these were to
be satisfactorily treated at home, a much improved and
extended system of district nurses would be needed.

MIDWIFERY

Most confinements in Austria are attended by midwives
at home or in special maternity homes. In Vienna three-

fourths of the births are stated to occur in maternity homes, only one-fourth in the mother's home. In other large towns maternity homes are common; while in rural districts some three-fourths of the births occur in the mother's own home. Even in maternity homes midwives attend normal parturitions, medical aid being invoked exceptionally.

Altogether in Austria there are some 5,000 midwives, or one to about 1,300 of the population. In 1925 the number of midwives in Vienna was 997, in 1926 it was 891, which is about 1 to 1,850 of total population, or 1·4 midwives to every 1,000 women of child-bearing ages.

Midwives generally dislike the institutional delivery of women, as it diminishes their private practice. The great increase of institutional provision is due largely to the high proportion of insured women, for whom and for the wives of insured men treatment in a lying-in home is a usual benefit of the society to which they belong. In Vienna some 60 per cent. of the population are included within the scope of social insurance. It is part of the official policy of the State to encourage maternity homes. In these homes maternal mortality is very low; and the insurance arrangements imply early registration of pregnancy, following on which prenatal care and supervision are exercised.

A law was passed in 1925 under which the regulations for the practice of midwifery have been revised. These contain detailed rules for the conduct of midwifery made by the Minister of Social Welfare of the Government. The midwives are supervised by the provincial councils. The county medical officer, acting for a subdivision of the province, is responsible for this work.

The midwife must call in a doctor in certain emergencies, the patient choosing her own doctor. If the patient is poor the communal (i.e. poor law) doctor is sent for. Any doctor sent for is under obligation to respond to an urgent call.

If an insured patient wishes to be confined at home, she can choose her own midwife, and the society to which she (or sometimes her husband) belongs must pay the midwife's fee according to a settled tariff.

It is legally compulsory for every commune or (in smaller areas) a combination of communes to appoint a midwife and to pay her a salary. This must be done if there are at least thirty to forty births in a year. The midwife is expected to supplement her small salary by private practice.

The encouragement of the use of maternity homes by insurance societies is a far-sighted policy, especially in view of the poverty and unfavourable home conditions of many of the insured. Both mothers and their infants gain in health by the superior care given in the maternity homes.

I visited a model lying-in home in Vienna conducted by a sickness insurance society which insures commercial employees and has a membership of 50,000. The institution is called Gynäkologisch-Geburtshilfliche Anstalt der Krankenkasse der Kaufmännisch Angestellten. This institution has seventy-four beds for insured women and the wives of insured men. There is a separate section for unmarried mothers. It has an obstetric and a gynæcological department. In the former no payment is required; in the latter, non-insured members of the family of the insured pay 5 Austrian shillings a day. On the obstetric side in three years five maternal deaths have occurred in connection with 1,800 births.

There is a carefully isolated section to which septic cases are admitted or transferred from the aseptic wards. There is a separate medical and nursing service for each section; and all the arrangements appeared to me to be ideal. The personnel is equal to one for every patient. The interne doctor attends each confinement; but the midwife conducts it.

To secure admission expectant mothers are registered in the fifth month of pregnancy. They are then required to attend monthly to ensure normal conditions or to ascertain complications promptly.

This institution was opened in 1926. It may be regarded

as a luxury establishment, in which the provision made—in every respect admirable—goes beyond what is necessary for essential safety and comfort. I was informed, however, that other maternity homes in Vienna come not far behind it in their arrangements.

The instillation of silver solution into the infants' eyes after birth is compulsory throughout Austria.

Midwives are trained in six special training-schools for midwives. These are maintained and administered by the Federal Government. The course of training lasts eighteen months, the first half of this time being devoted to training in obstetrics, the second half to child hygiene and infant welfare work. At the State University Hospital in Vienna, which has 3,500 maternity cases in the year, fourteen student midwives reside in the hospital during two periods of a fortnight, and are continuously on duty during this time, though they do not undertake deliveries. Antenatal work is taught on a large scale.

Puerperal Mortality.—The national statistics show unsatisfactory conditions. Infant mortality is high. The national birth-rate in 1922–25 was 22·2 per 1,000 of population. In 1927 it was 18·5, that of Vienna being 11·5 per 1,000 total births, including the stillborn. The proportion of illegitimate to total births in the same year was 25·2 per cent. for Austria as a whole, and 23·7 per cent. for Vienna. The death-rate from puerperal sepsis alone in 1927 was 2·07 per 1,000 total births for Austria, and 3·91 for Vienna. The excess of puerperal sepsis in Vienna suggests an excessive proportion of abortions in that city. (Figures calculated from data, *Mitteilungen des Volkgesundheitsamtes*, Heft 11 and 12, for 1928.)

MATERNITY AND CHILD WELFARE

For insured women, and usually for the wives of insured men, an allowance is given for six weeks before and after confinement (see page 213) and a breast-feeding benefit is given for the first twelve weeks after confinement, if the mother nurses her baby. In Vienna breast-feeding during the first three months is stated to be continued for at least 90 per cent. of infants.

Mothers (see page 202) are most often confined in maternity homes in Vienna, and in these homes puerperal sepsis is stated to be rare. The sepsis figures for the whole city, as shown in the preceding section, are unfavourable. There are both municipal and insurance maternity homes.

There is no complete system of home visitation of infants, though this is done in connection with some special institutions. This great lack is owing, in part at least, to the divided forces concerned in helping mothers and their infants.

These are—

    (1) Municipal and other authorities,
    (2) Voluntary organisations, and
    (3) Insurance societies.

Local authorities concern themselves chiefly with neglected and deserted children, and with the problems of illegitimacy; and the normal child—whose mother needs guidance and help—is apt to be neglected. The gap is to some extent filled up for the mothers and infants in insured households by the clinics and dispensaries provided by insurance societies. But these, although they are a great boon, do not provide for home visitation by health visitors or public health nurses. This visitation, and the influences arising from it, forms an important measure for securing improvement of child hygiene.

The rate of infant mortality varies greatly in different parts of Austria, as does also the mortality in the second and third year of life. The national figures show very excessive child mortality in the parts of Austria near Bavaria, in which very young children are fed with meat; and in other parts of Austria infants are given poppy-seed extract to keep them quiet. In Carinthia 40 per cent. of infants are illegitimate, and their death-rate is very excessive.

The statistics kindly given me by Dr. Siegfried Rosenfeld, the chief of the National Bureau of Vital Statistics, show that around and in Vienna infant mortality is relatively low. In Vienna it was—

80·0 per 1,000 births in 1927, and
82·5 per 1,000 births in 1928.

In Burgenland it was 158·7 and 157·4 in the same two years. This part of present Austria was formerly part of Hungary.

An example of excellent maternity and child welfare work (in addition to that mentioned on page 203) is given by the Reichanstalt für Mütter- und Säuglingsfürsorge in Wien, which I visited.

This institution is entirely supported by the State, except for payments made by parents, which are lenient, and payments made by insurance societies, which send patients here at a fixed charge. Cases of bad metabolism in infants and very young children are admitted; as are also infants with their mothers in whom breast-feeding is failing. There is a wet-nursing department. All medical conditions in young children are admissible, including tuberculous patients. There are about 125 beds, including the beds for mothers, who are sometimes transferred direct to this institution from maternity homes.

There is an infant consultation clinic attached to the hospital. A large proportion of children are transferred through the director of this hospital to Alpine and seaside convalescent homes. It may be added here that similar work is done on a very large scale both by municipal authorities and insurance societies : and, as Austria now has no seaboard, a mutual arrangement has been made with German authorities, in virtue of which German children come to Alpine resorts in Austria and Austrian children go to marine resorts in North Germany. Several houses are also rented on the Adriatic seacoast. Some 35,000 children are sent yearly to these summer resorts, the funds being derived from private charity and from municipal, State, and insurance sources. Parents are expected to contribute when they can, and often pay entirely for their children in these vacations,

Attached to this institution is an interesting nursing training-school, for nurses who will be babies' nurses or public-health nurses in child welfare work (Fürsorgerinnen). The course of training lasts for one year. The syllabus is excellent, including not only physiology and anatomy and pediatrics, but also elementary obstetrics and pathology, social diseases, and social laws and insurance. Forty students are admitted each year. They pay for their board, but the training is provided at the expense of the State. Most of the nurses thus trained go out as Fürsorgerinnen, especially for rural districts.

In Austria there are about 475 "well baby centres". These are in charge of part-time doctors, who in cities and larger towns are specialists; in the rural districts the consultations are held by general practitioners. There are attached to each of these centres one to two Fürsorgerinnen, who assist the doctor in his work, and make also home visits. They undertake "follow-up" work, and persuade mothers to come to the centres as early as possible after the infant's birth. Midwives are under an obligation to notify each birth attended by them, within forty-eight hours after confinement, to the local registrar or to the burgomaster's office. From these sources the Fürsorgerin obtains the information enabling her to call at the homes of recently delivered mothers.

School Medical Inspection

Outside Vienna and the capital cities of its nine provinces there is but little medical inspection of school children. In Vienna there are about 120,000 children aged six to fourteen in its elementary schools, and there are forty-nine school doctors. The chief school medical officer is a whole-time officer; the remainder give a few hours daily to their work, each doctor having allotted to him a share of the 556 elementary school buildings in Vienna. I was unable to judge whether this arrangement is satisfactory. The routine procedure is a complete physical examination of each scholar soon after admission to school, and twice afterwards.

Defective children are more frequently examined. School nurses (Fürsorgerinnen) do some home visiting. The same nurses are concerned also in child welfare work.

No treatment of defects is undertaken by the school doctors, but cases are referred to the private doctor, to the insurance society to which the parent belongs, or to a hospital. If a child has adenoids, for instance, a notice is sent to the parents, and it is expected that the private doctor will act, or that the patient will be taken to a hospital.

This does not mean, as might appear, that the child is necessarily neglected. In the majority of instances he belongs to a family the head of which is insured; and commonly (not always) this means that the child is entitled to treatment by the Krankenkassen. Most societies have specialists for these diseases, for eye corrections, and for various other children's ailments, at their ambulatoria.

The only treatment carried out on behalf of the municipality is for dental diseases. There are eleven school dental clinics in Vienna, all with modern equipment, in which whole-time dental officers are employed. All children in the schools are examined, and all those found to need it are treated whose parents are not well-to-do, or who cannot receive treatment through insurance societies.

Routine lessons are given by the dental officers on dental hygiene, and each scholar is expected to bring with him a toothbrush for class teaching and demonstration!

In the provinces school medical inspection is legally compulsory; but, except in large towns, little or nothing is done. An attempt was made to impose the duty of school-inspection on the communal doctor without additional salary. In a few places this work has succeeded; sometimes, it has been suggested, as a means of obtaining private practice.

Some large industrial firms, like Krupps, have established school medical services in the districts in which their works are situated.

TUBERCULOSIS

Dr. Rosenfeld, the Government's statistician, informed
me that in 1926 the death-rate in Austria from all forms of
tuberculosis was 16·6, and in 1926 it was 17·14 per 10,000
inhabitants. It is highest in towns. In Vienna in 1911–13 it

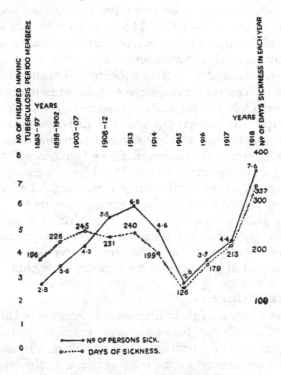

INSURANCE EXPERIENCE OF TUBERCULOSIS BEFORE &
DURING THE WAR. (ROSENFELD)
IN VIENNA AND LOWER AUSTRIA.

was 29·8 per 10,000, and it became much higher during
the Great War.

Insurance societies are greatly interested, especially
financially, in the tuberculosis problem. From a special
report by Dr. Rosenfeld I take the figures on which the
above curves are based. They summarise the experience
of the Krankenkassen of Vienna and Lower Austria during

a series of years up to 1919. Evidently a large part of the funds of the insurance societies have been swallowed up by tuberculosis. This loss greatly increased in the war years.

In 1928 there were 68 tuberculosis dispensaries in Austria, of which 24 were organised by communal authorities, 37 by private associations, 3 by industrial enterprises, and 4 by sickness insurance societies. This number does not include the special clinics of various insurance societies at their respective central consulting-rooms.

The official and voluntary tuberculosis dispensaries are regarded as centres for diagnosis and for work in preventive medicine. Only exceptionally is treatment given on a small scale, especially in rural districts. The dispensary serves also as a clearing station, at which arrangements for institutional residential treatment are made. Some "follow-up" work is done by Fürsorgerinnen attached to these dispensaries.

There are many well-managed sanatoria. The municipality of Vienna has 2,000 beds for consumptives.

On a general review it must be said that very inadequate national work is being done for the prevention and treatment of tuberculosis; and that this defect is perhaps the weakest part of the work of the insurance societies.

Venereal Diseases

Great increase of these diseases was experienced after the Great War, and they became widely spread in rural districts to an extent not previously known. These diseases have always been treated in the general and special hospitals of great towns; and in recent years the Insurance Krankenkassen have special clinics for them. Patients with these diseases are treated on the same basis as for other diseases, and receive their sickness benefits.

Since the war venereal disease dispensaries have been opened in each of the nine provinces of Austria, including Vienna itself as one of these. Altogether there are about thirty of these dispensaries. They are known as Abend-Ambulatoria from the usual time of the clinic. There are separate hours for female patients. Specialists conduct these clinics. They are open to all comers, free treatment being given. Insurance Krankenkassen encourage attendance at these clinics, and supply neo-salvarsan to all insured persons suffering from syphilis who apply for it. This is taken by the patient to the Abend-Ambulatorium, the specialist then undertaking its administration. It has not been found that the ambulatoria interfere greatly with private medical practice, as many patients do not like the possibilities of publicity associated with delays in the ambulatorium waiting-rooms. The work of the ambulatoria is carried out under the supervision of the Provincial Health Departments at the cost of the State.

In Vienna since 1924 a special effort to reduce congenital syphilis has been made, which has exceptional interest. It is freely announced in public places and by circulars, etc., that any pregnant woman who, up to the fourth month of pregnancy, attends a special clinic in order that a Wasserman test may be made will, if found to be syphilitic, and if she is destitute and not a member of an insurance society will, even if not syphilitic, receive a cash benefit of 10 Austrian shillings during each of four weeks after confinement.

SOCIAL INSURANCES

Austria has a system of social insurance which includes sickness, accident, invalidity, unemployment, and (for a section of the population) old age. Old age insurance is in force for persons who are employed in offices, banks, etc., and who receive a monthly or a quarterly salary. It does not yet apply to workmen on a weekly wage, although the law making this extension compulsory has already been passed, and will come into force when the financial position of Austria permits.

So far as sickness insurance is concerned, the insured are classified in two categories: (a) manual workers in receipt of a weekly wage, and (b) employees whose work is not manual, employed as clerks, typists, shop assistants, etc., and who are paid a monthly salary. These two categories are treated separately in the Insurance Acts.

Commonly they are included in societies or Krankenkassen which deal with only one of the two classes.

In some societies—at present mostly societies for employees—the sickness insurance includes medical treatment for the entire family of the insured, in others this is not so; and the medical profession, as voiced by its organisations (see statement on p. 221) is in general opposition to the extension for medical treatment of sickness insurance to the families of the insured. A recent enactment enables insurance societies to do this.

In accordance with the law, insurance societies must be occupational or localised in their distribution. This avoids much of the complexities of administration and excessive secretarial expenses occurring in the English system. As a rule the worker has a choice between two societies, and often this means a choice between a society of a socialist and one of anti-socialistic tendencies.

The total number of manual labourers and employees embraced by sickness insurance in Austria is 1,800,000 persons. This figure means only the insured themselves; members of the families of the insured number roughly 2,500,000 persons. There are, therefore, about 4,300,000 persons in Austria partaking of the benefits of sickness insurance, or 65·8 per cent. of the total population. This high proportion means that social insurance has extended into social classes not usually included. It relates to employed persons generally without any limitation of income. Thus a bank director or manager is insured because he receives a salary, and the same holds good for all municipal and State officials. The medical staff of the Ministry of Social Welfare are insured for medical attendance, 2 to 3 per cent. of their salary being deducted for this purpose.

The benefits obtainable under sickness insurance include a cash allowance during the insured person's incapacitating illness for a period not exceeding seventy-eight weeks; free obstetric help for the insured woman or the wife of an insured man; free medical treatment, including the cost of drugs, etc., by the insurance doctor; also certain additional benefits for mothers as set out in the following paragraphs. The benefits also include, when needed, hospital treatment in the third class. Hospital patients are divided into three classes in accordance with the quality of accommodation required; professional men commonly pay an additional sum to be transferred to smaller wards.

Sickness Insurance.—Perhaps the best idea can be given of the Austrian system of sickness insurance by an account of the activities of a relatively small Viennese society, whose central institution I visited. This society caters for labourers in commercial enterprises and trades, as, for instance, industrial car-drivers, etc. It has about 15,000

CONTRIBUTIONS AND BENEFITS OF THE ARBEITER-KRANKEN-KASSE DES GREMIUMS DER WIENER KAUFMANNSCHAFT

(Insurance Society of Workers in Commercial Enterprises)

A. Wages and Contributions (in shillings)

Classification of Workers according to Wage	Daily Wage	Weekly Wage	Weekly Contributions to the Society (Shillings)			
			For Sickness	For Unemployment [1]	Other Payments [2]	Total Payments
I	1·13	6·77	0·54	0·40	0·59	1·53
II	1·39	8·35	0·63	0·48	0·63	1·74
III	1·73	10·37	0·78	0·58	0·73	2·09
IV	1·87	11·23	0·90	0·68	0·78	2·36
V	2·40	14·40	1·05	0·78	0·88	2·71
VI	3·00	18·00	1·35	1·02	1·00	3·37
VII	3·60	21·60	1·65	1·24	1·19	4·08
VIII	4·80	28·80	2·10	1·58	1·40	5·08
IX	6·00	36·00	2·40	1·80	1·54	5·74
X	over 6·00	over 36·00	2·70	2·02	1·69	6·41

[1] Two-thirds paid by employer, one-third paid by worker.
[2] For sickness, for administration of the society, and for old age, the contributions by employers and employed are equal. The contributions for sanatoria, convalescent homes, etc., are made two-thirds by employers and one-third by employed.

B. Sickness Benefits

Classification of Workers according to Wages (see A)	Daily Allowance in Shillings during Illness				Daily Allowance in Shillings	
	During the first Four Weeks	After Fourth Week	After Twentieth Week	After Fifty-second Week	In the Six Weeks before and Six Weeks following Childbirth	Rest Premium (Daily) Twelfth to Twenty-second Week
I	0·86	0·90	1·00	1·08	0·86	0·43
II	1·00	1·10	1·20	1·25	1·00	0·50
III	1·24	1·40	1·50	1·55	1·24	0·62
IV	1·44	1·60	1·70	1·80	1·44	0·72
V	1·70	1·80	2·00	2·10	1·70	0·85
VI	2·00	2·20	2·40	2·50	2·00	1·00
VII	2·40	2·60	2·80	3·00	2·40	1·20
VIII	3·00	3·20	3·40	3·50	3·00	1·50
IX	3·60	3·60	3·60	3·60	3·60	1·80
X	4·20	4·20	4·20	4·20	4·20	2·10

There is an allowance of 30 shillings for the midwife's fee, and a sum varying from 50 shillings in class I to 210 shillings in class X for funeral expenses.

In addition, for members of an insured family—not themselves separately insured—there is the same allowance for a midwife, a daily allowance of half a shilling as a rest premium, and an allowance for cost of funerals, varying from 20 to 50 shillings according to age.

The closeness of relationship between wages, sickness contributions, and cash benefits (during the fifth to the twentieth week of sickness) is better shown in the diagram on facing page, in which the amounts for the first class of workers in each curve are represented as one hundred, and for other classes of workers in proportion.

members. It is called the Central Institute for the Insurance of Workers in Commercial Enterprises (Krankenkasse des Gremiums der Wiener Kaufmannschaft). The premiums payable for sickness insurance in this society are shown in tables at foot of page 213 and above.

It will be seen that the insured are classified under ten headings according to their wages. The premium paid is a sum which is fixed by legislation. It is not an exact percentage of the worker's wages, equal for all wages. As seen in the diagram, contributions do not run strictly parallel with wages. The premiums payable by employers and employed

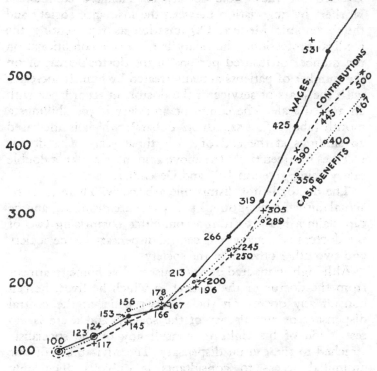

Comparative Course of Contributions (Premiums),
Cash Benefits, and Wages.

and the financial benefits for the employed are set out in the preceding table.

We are chiefly concerned, however, with the medical benefits. Each insured patient receives complete medical attendance in sickness as part of his or her benefit. This is given in the society cited above, so far as concerns domiciliary attendance and consultations at the doctor's office, by a doctor who receives a fixed salary for his work in a prescribed district; and the patient is limited to this doctor for home treatment. The salary paid to the doctor is fixed for the whole society of Viennese commercial workers by negotiation between the insurance society and the Economic Medical Organisation as representing the medical profession. The salary is not made conditional on the number of insured persons in the doctor's area, or on the number of patients actually treated by him. It increases with the years of service of the doctor, in accordance with an agreed scale. The commencing salary is 300 shillings a month (about £8 15s., or 42 dollars), which is increased 20 shillings at the end of every three years. The doctor receives fourteen times the above amount in a year, a double salary being given in July and December.

The doctor is not dismissible arbitrarily. There must be actual misdemeanour on his part to secure dismissal, and he can claim a hearing from a committee comprising two of the doctors engaged at the central dispensary of the society and two other officials of the society.

Although an insured person must receive home treatment from the doctor of the district in which he lives, he can consult any doctor on the society's panel at the central dispensary or ambulatory of the society, and there is no restriction of his right to consult any of the specialists attached to the central dispensary. The advisability of this unlimited access to consultants is dubious. The only exception made is as to the use of X-rays, which can be prescribed only by the dispensary consultants.

The patient receives hospital treatment when required during a period of twenty-eight days as part of his benefit. If more prolonged treatment in a hospital is needed, then the patient must pay, or he is paid for by the province (Vienna is a separate province of Austria) as part of its subvention to hospitals.

The cost of administration in this society amounts to 10·5 per cent. of its total expenditure. The society gives no family financial insurance, except to the extent indicated in the table. It gives medical attendance to the family. Such inclusive family insurance for medical treatment of the insured person's family is common, but is not compulsory as yet. Each society chooses whether family benefits shall be included in its scheme.

If an insured person is dissatisfied with his doctor, the matter is referred to the chief consulting physician at the dispensary. Most disputes arise when the doctor thinks, but the patient denies, that he is fit for work. From the consultant's opinion the insured may appeal further to a committee of Trustees, a jury composed of equal numbers of representatives of the society and of the insured. This is the final court of appeal.

Recently the society has appointed controllers to supervise domiciliary benefits. They are not doctors. Each patient is visited at least once during his illness, at an unexpected hour, to ensure that he is not engaged in some wage-earning occupation. The same difficulty as to consumptive patients is experienced as in England. On medical grounds these often should have some light occupation.

In some larger societies—some of them may have half a million labouring members—medical controllers are also employed.

At the central dispensary of the above society are admirable offices for consultation and treatment for conditions requiring special skill, and each department is manned by doctors having skill in their own part of medicine. I saw the separate consulting-rooms devoted to—

Internal medicine;
Surgery, including a separate operating theatre for minor surgery;
Pathological diagnoses;
Eye diseases;
Throat, ear, and nose diseases,
X-ray diagnosis and treatment;
Artificial light treatment;
Gynæcological treatment;
Dental treatment.

The specialists at work here are paid the sum of 320 shillings a month (about £9 5s., or 45 dollars) for an hour's service every weekday.

In the eye clinic insured persons receive any spectacles (including plain frames) that may be prescribed, but must pay for gold frames if they want them!

Artificial-light treatment can be recommended by a district doctor, but is only given when approved by the chief medical officer of the institute.

The gynæcological department is required for insured women, among whom are shop-assistants, etc.

The dentists carry out extractions and fillings, and supply dentures. No additional payment is required for dentures, which are supplied in all cases in which they are regarded as necessary for health.

I received the impression that, although the provision for general and special medical treatment at the dispensary was admirable, excessive waiting for consultation was associated with the system, as in the out-patient departments of some voluntary hospitals in England.

The payment of the doctor per insured person on his personal list or panel is unknown in Austria. At the central dispensaries or ambulatories the doctor is paid for each attendance of one to three hours, as already indicated, under a contract between the Krankenkasse and the doctor.

For domiciliary attendance or office consultations (at the doctor's house) two systems are in operation:—

(1) As in the society instanced above, the doctors are districted. This holds good for societies in which manual workers are insured. A doctor is appointed for each district by the society on the basis of knowledge of the approximate number of insured in that district belonging to the society, and is paid a monthly salary for this work. This is the same system as holds generally throughout Hungary. Sometimes the doctor is overworked, sometimes he has little work; but his salary is fixed.

He is not expected to devote his whole time to his insurance patients. In the above-mentioned society his salary begins at 300 shillings a month; in country districts it may be 250 shillings, an amount which tempts young doctors, and it may not increase beyond 500 to 700 shillings a month. In sparsely populated districts there is a "point system" providing a fixed addition in accordance with distances to be travelled in visiting patients.

(2) For societies which insure non-manual workers a different system is commonly adopted. The insured person by the rules of the society is free to consult any doctor in private practice, whose fees he must pay. He then obtains a statement from the doctor of his choice stating the number of consultations and visits made, and he can claim from the society payment for each of these—or only a portion of it —according to the fixed tariff of the society.

(3) A modification of the second system is sometimes adopted. Some societies insuring employees (defined as on p. 211) employ doctors on a direct contract basis, in which payment is made by the society in accordance with the amount of services rendered, and not directly by the patient. The doctor of the patient's personal choice enters on special forms issued by the society the number of consultations or visits made with each patient. These forms are sent periodically to the central office of the insurance company, are revised by the clerical staff of the society, and payment is then made in accordance with a scale agreed on between the society and the Economic Medical Association.

In these latter societies consultations with the experts at the ambulatory are only permitted with the consent of the patient's private doctor; but the insured person has an appeal to the society against any veto of the doctor. Obviously this difficulty will arise chiefly when there is doubt as to the patient's fitness for work.

Outside Vienna it is not so easy to obtain expert consultations, except in some larger towns; but as the population of Vienna is 1,850,000, and that of Austria only about 6,700,000, the above description holds good for over a fourth of the entire population—probably much more, as the proportion of insured is highest in industrial centres.

It is difficult to obtain independent testimony of the preponderant judgment of patients, of doctors, and of insurance societies on these various methods of contract medical practice. I have been fortunate in securing the appended statement representing the views of the organised medical profession in Austria on the working of the present sickness insurance system, and on the general attitude of the medical profession to the conditions of medical service in this insurance, for which I am deeply indebted to Dr. Weinlaender. It will be seen that it is far from favourable, although the impossibility of retracing steps already taken or of immediate improvement in the conditions of medical services is recognised.

The observations made on the public health medical services reveal also an attitude which is fairly general in Europe. So long as treatment is not given in these dispensary services, well and good; but when, as not infrequently happens, this rule is not respected, the province of the private medical practitioner is regarded as having been invaded. This attitude does not, it appears to me, make adequate allowance for cases of minor ailments which would remain untreated if not dealt with at Child Hygiene Consultations and School Clinics, nor with such conditions as defects of eye-refraction, chronic otorrhœa, adenoids, etc., of which the same may often be said. Nor in regard to venereal diseases does this attitude allow for the supreme importance of giving early and adequate treatment without a trace of inhibitory influences. But these are general points to be discussed in another volume.

The attitude of insurance patients sometimes is one of partial distrust of the doctor, as being in the employment of the insurance society, and therefore under an implied obligation to economise, especially on drugs, not altogether to the advantage of the patient. When there is no choice of domiciliary doctor, the patient may even prefer to pay the fee of a private practitioner. This sometimes happens.

Reform is called for, also, in regard to the occasional protracted waiting of patients both at doctors' offices and at the ambulatories.

The bureaucratic administration of insurance societies is a frequent source of complaint. There is apparently an insuperable tendency to increase and complicate the machinery of administration. This is not limited to any country or any official or quasi-official organisation. The doctors object to this, because a large share of their valuable professional time is occupied in filling up forms; and patients fret at the complexities almost necessarily associated with the granting of weekly monetary benefits on a large scale. Only a statesmanlike master-mind in administration can reduce these sources of friction, of waste of time and money, to the minimum consistent with economical efficiency.

MEMORANDUM ON THE INFLUENCE OF PUBLIC HEALTH WORK ON THE PRIVATE PRACTICE OF THE MEDICAL PROFESSION IN AUSTRIA

By Georg Weinlaender, M.D.,
President of the Economic Medical Society of Vienna,
Vice-President of the National Association of Austrian
     Medical Societies,
President of the Economic Society of Dentists in Vienna.

Among the questions asked me by Sir Arthur Newsholme, the most important is the one concerning the influence of public compulsory sickness insurance on the professional work of the medical practitioner. Apart from the general effect of these arrangements, to which I will return later, we must bear in mind that in Austria, in consequence of the unhappy result of the war and the downfall of the Empire, together with the loss in value of the currency, there are two essential matters which are specially damaging to the medical profession, viz. the flooding of the remaining territory of the State with the members of the intelligentsia, especially medical men, resulting in a superabundance of the profession: and the impoverishment of the whole population, especially of the middle classes, who were formerly the mainstay of the medical profession. Even without social insurance there would be a serious reduction in the earnings of Austrian medical men; but these earnings have been still further reduced by the inclusion of nearly 80 per cent. of the population in such insurance.

The influence of social insurance on the conditions of medical practice is affected by the way in which the medical service is rendered, in regard to the system adopted and the amounts paid. There are two methods adopted in Austria: fixed salaries of medical men with a right to a pension, or free choice of doctors. The fixed salaries system is stoutly opposed by the majority of medical men, as it cuts out most of them from practice for the insured part of the population.

The appointed doctors complain of the loss of their freedom, their dependence upon the Kassen managers, excessive administrative certificates, especially as regards fitness for work, and dissatisfaction with the purely medical work, which often becomes stereotyped, and only forms a fraction of their actual work.

The insured are to a great extent dissatisfied with the medical attendance supplied by the Kasse, as they regard the Kassen doctor as appointed to serve the interests of the Kasse and not the patient's interests, an official and not the doctor, who has the confidence of his patient. Patients, therefore, very often seek other medical men, whom they pay out of their own pockets, and make use of the Kassen doctor only to get certificates.

The doctor is deprived of freedom, has little interest in the sick, and contents himself in most cases with purely outside routine, sending every difficult case to the specialist or to the public ambulatories, which in this way are burdened with expenses for which the State has already paid in the form of subventions for social insurance. The overwhelming majority of the Austrian medical profession—except the small portion who are Social Democrats, and who favour the officialisation of the medical profession by law, and the larger portion who find themselves in fixed and well-paid situations, or are given work by the Kassen whereby free expression of opinions is naturally at least reduced and influenced—are more or less opposed to social insurance, because it results in a much circumscribed medical practice, because the direct relationship between the doctor and the patients is spoilt by the intervention of the Kasse as paymaster of medical work, and because the doctors in practice are out of patience with the many unsatisfactory consequences to them of insurance, in the shape of unnecessary demands for medical help and sick pay, without any recompense to themselves in the way of better results or obvious improvement in the public health. The circumstances that the Krankenkassen determine the nature and extent of medical help, that this duty is entrusted to them and not to any other pecuniarily disinterested party, that the doctors never have a word to say in decisions affecting the medical care of the insured (as is the case in Austria),

discredit social insurance (so far as it consists in the care of the
sick) most seriously in the eyes of a majority of the Austrian
medical profession.

A further unsatisfactory feature is the insufficient payments
for services rendered, which doubtless arises in part from the
limited means of the Kassen and the largely unnecessary payments (to patients) demanded and made.

The widely regretted overtreatment, so far as it is the fault
of the doctor, is only partly the result of greed (on their part)
and results mainly because the doctor, in consequence of his
dependence on both sides, is not in a position to oppose unjusti-
fiable demands. The doctor in such cases is "the whipping-boy
between the two parties".

All things considered, after making full allowance for the
benefits of social insurance, especially in catastrophes, in serious
long-continued illness, and in necessary operations, it cannot be
denied that the present form of such insurance has serious
defects, and especially that it damages the ethics of the medical
profession and the quality of medical services.

Scientific work finds its reward neither in the gratitude of the
patients, the recognition of the Kasse, nor in higher salaries;
while, on the other hand, the careless routine-pursuing doctor,
who knows best how to avoid conflicts with either side, is the
most successful.

The consequences of such a state of affairs are easy to see. It
is a question whether future developments in social insurance,
so far as it concerns the curative part of medical work, will not
result in pure accident insurance and full independence of the
medical profession; as in this department, so far, abuses lie
open to the day.

Decidedly simpler and less damaging to the professional
activity of the medical man are the other benefits of public care
(Fürsorge), such as advice to mothers, the care of infants, tuberculosis, sexual disorders, and school doctoring. All of these
measures can, and will, in the course of time, prove themselves
a wonderful blessing, by raising the general health of the people;
and this without damaging the medical profession, if the fundamental condition has been arrived at that in all these measures
no individual treatment is given, but only prophylactic advice.
Doubtless it must be admitted that in these departments the
officials and other persons concerned go beyond their province,
and that many sick persons seek help at the Fürsorge stations for
conditions which necessarily involve medical treatment, resulting
in a heavy inroad on medical practice. *All the more is this the
case where, as in Austria, there are neither legal regulations against
applications by those with means for free treatment and advice, nor*

condemnation on the part of public opinion of such abuses, which might form a dam against their evil consequences. The Austrian Economic Medical Association wages incessant warfare against these repeated abuses of public welfare work (Fürsorge), also often against medical men in practice who draw personal economic benefits from this state of affairs, not only in their official capacity, but also by increase of their private practice. Very often, however, the medical man is not even paid; and this is the worse, because the doctors with such duties are very often compelled, especially under present-day unfortunate economic conditions, to get payment in other ways, to the great detriment of the whole medical profession. If from the commencement of the welfare movement the condition agreed upon with the medical profession had been strictly adhered to, that medical treatment was to be excluded from welfare stations, and that these were to be kept entirely for prophylactic advice, not only would no damage have been done to medical men in this practice and in general respects, but the economic prospects of the profession would have been improved by the establishment of a new and important branch of work. The greatest care was taken in avoiding fundamental errors from the very beginning of the public welfare movement, especially on the part of the medical representatives, who in this respect could not help being very distrustful, since with the best will in the world on the part of the persons concerned there are great dangers grounded in the character of humanity. *For every insurance and every welfare movement lends itself fundamentally to misuse,* and the most ideal institution or the most ideal management is scarcely in a position to shut abuses out entirely. The position of medical men in Austrian and German social insurance is fundamentally bad in this respect and in need of reform, because the medical representatives have omitted to recognise the danger in time and to prevent it.

It is only to be hoped for the German and Austrian medical men that a revolution in public opinion will eventually take place through the example of other countries, who, it is to be hoped, are learning from our evil experiences and those of our German colleagues, and who will testify that other ways work well, and a good social insurance can be carried out without enslaving a free medical profession. If so we shall succeed with iron energy in preventing the complete enslavement of the profession. The welfare movement in Austria, whose consequences to the medical profession I have sketched in large outlines in the foregoing paragraphs, omitting, therefore, many details of the separate matters requiring attention, is in a bad way because there is no systematic organisation of the various interests, viz. the State, the autonomous Krankenkassen, and private charitable societies, etc. In consequence, they largely overlap, and even if not actually opposed to one another, do not properly co-operate. *A tuberculosis welfare centre run by a Krankenkasse is an absurdity, so long as the members of the same family belong to different Kassen which are not working together at the same time.* And that is the case with us. The whole welfare movement belongs to the State, and medical men should be appointed to it who have no private practice. This would bring about a much better relationship between welfare centres and the medical profession. Specially difficult is the work in maternal advice centres and infant care centres, concerning which complaints that treatment is given are particularly frequent. This would naturally be the case. As regards the fight against sexual disorders, the question of the maintenance of professional secrecy is a common stone of contention, which prejudices the good results of these measures, and gives rise to opposition on the part of the doctors. The medical control of school-children should give least occasion for opposition by the medical profession, because here for the most part healthy children are controlled, and this compulsorily and not in the shape of voluntary choice, as in the public welfare centres, where mostly people go who already have more or less reason to feel out of health, or suspect the need of treatment for a coming illness.

In fact, at least half of the people who seek advice at the welfare centres belong here, already a priori from the recommendation of the medical officer as regards treatment. At the inauguration of a welfare centre stress should more and more be laid publicly upon the fact that diagnosis takes the first place, and that welfare centres are *not places for treatment*, since amongst us the contrary idea is widely accepted.

If in the foregoing I have mainly criticised, it is only right in conclusion to state that social insurance in Austria has given a means of livelihood, even if under difficult conditions, to a section of the medical profession who otherwise would have had nothing to live upon, since a majority of the wholly impoverished population, including the middle classes, would not seek private medical help. This purely economic consideration, which, however, must be doubly opposed in offering services, and which to a great extent is equivalent to robbery of both health and working capacity, naturally makes no change in the fundamental injuries which were set forth in the foregoing, as regards deterioration of the ethics of the profession and of the quality of their services, through the deprival of the medical man's independence and personal responsibility.

CHAPTER VII

SWITZERLAND[1]

PRELIMINARY SUMMARY

Each of the twenty-five cantons of this small country has almost complete home rule, and many variations of administration on medical and hygienic problems are found.

Some measure of unification is supplied by the federal grants given in aid of anti-tuberculosis work, sickness insurance, etc.

There is much active anti-tuberculosis work. Tuberculosis dispensaries, as in France, avoid the domain of the private medical practitioner.

Many interesting experiments in social insurance are found in different cantons. Compulsory sickness and accident insurance for the whole of Switzerland was rejected on referendum.

The Federal Government subsidises voluntary sickness societies which fulfil certain conditions.

In all such societies (*caisses*) the insured person can choose his own doctor within reasonable limits.

Insurance doctors are paid by tariffs based on the number and character of attendances.

In some cantons there is compulsory sickness insurance, its extent varying in different cantons. In the canton Vaud parents are required to insure for the provision of medical treatment for their children during school-life. In Bâle the majority of the total population is under sickness insurance.

In some cantons mothers receive monetary or other assistance in parturition and during lactation.

In connection with the salt monopoly the sale of iodised salt is compulsory in some cantons.

Attempts at controlling alcoholism have met with little success.

[1] Date of investigation, March 1929.

GENERAL CONDITIONS

The medico-hygienic problems of Switzerland present many features worthy of study. Although this country forms only a small patch on the map of Europe, it comprises within it twenty-five almost completely self-governing areas (cantons), which have utilised their organised social life in varied forms presenting many special features.

The analogy between Switzerland and the United States of America strikes even the casual observer. The U.S.A. is a great and Switzerland a small country: but the smaller country probably presents as great variations in enactments and in methods of public administration and social activities as are manifested in the forty-eight sovereign United States. The smaller country comprises three races in its population, with a steady persistence of three chief languages; while in the United States of America, although centres of Italian, of German, and of Slavonic-speaking peoples persist, unification, in language at least, is in rapid progress.

Both countries owe their local autonomy to historic causes; for the cantons and the States existed before the Helvetian Confederation and the Federal Government of the United States came into being. This local independence has great value, and perhaps greater drawbacks when public health and great social problems are concerned. Thus the control of alcohol has caused, and is causing, much embarrassment in both countries. Public health administration in both countries would advance more rapidly if there were organised a minimum order of uniformity, with full freedom to experiment and extend beyond the stage of minimum equality of accomplishment. And in the problems of social insurance in which both countries are interested, and in which Switzerland has advanced greatly in individual cantons, national uniformity of legislation and of administration is almost indispensable for success and continuity in any scheme that may be proposed.

The census population of Switzerland in 1920 was 3,880,320, and in 1927 about 107,000 more than this. It comprises twenty-five cantons within the Helvetian Federation

(Confederation *jurée* or Eidgenossenschaft). Its population presents three main groups: the growers of cattle of the Alpine valleys, the peasants of the plains, and the industrial workers in the towns.

GOVERNMENT

Each canton has its own separate constitution, and the Confederation is limited in its oversight and control. Thus there are twenty-five complete States, only limited by the functions belonging to the Federal constitution. The extent of these is somewhat doubtful. The Federal Government can make general legislation as to the control of epidemic diseases, tuberculosis, and syphilis.

The Federal Parliament consists of representatives from the whole of Switzerland, forming the National Council, which is elected on a system of proportional representation for three years; and a second chamber, the States Council, comprising two members from each canton. When the two Chambers have agreed on legislation, this is subject to *facultative referendum* to the whole people, if 30,000 citizens demand this within ninety days.

The cantons have a similar organisation, except that there is only one chamber. In most cantons legislation, and sometimes also regulations, are required to be submitted to the direct vote of the people (*obligatory referendum*). In all the cantons a certain number of citizens have the "right of popular initiative", i.e. of proposing new laws.

The executive work of the Federal Government is carried out by a Federal Council (Conseil Fédéral) of seven members, elected for three years by the two Federal Chambers meeting as the Federal Assembly. The Federal Council constitutes the Government, each Federal Councillor being in charge of one of the seven Federal Departments of work. One of these is the Federal Department of the Interior, comprising in its activities the public health service. The Federal Council is responsible to the Federal Assembly, which each year appoints one of its seven members as President of the Confederation.

Each Cantonal Council delegates its power to a State Council (Conseil d'État). There are usually from five to nine cantonal departments in a canton. Each of these has its separate health service. There is a further division into districts, with a prefect to each district; and, in addition, districts are subdivided into communes, governed by a syndic or mayor.

The arrangements thus indicated imply extreme decentralisation of medico-hygienic official work; and this gives the opportunity for study of very varied methods of administration on a small scale.

VITAL STATISTICS

The Federal Health Bureau was established in 1890, and empowered to collect statistics: and in each canton the registrar of vital statistics is subject to the supervision of the federal authorities. A confidential method of death certification has been adopted, in which it is arranged for the medical part of the certificate to go direct to the central bureau, thus maintaining medical secrecy. The vital statistics of Switzerland are exceptionally trustworthy. Of the total deaths, only from 3 to 4 per cent. fail to be medically attested.

MEDICAL ORGANISATION

The regulations for the canton of Zurich illustrate the general position. The practice of medicine by unqualified persons is forbidden; but qualified doctors from neighbouring cantons may practise in Zurich without a special "patent", provided that reciprocal permission is given. Under the Zurich Medical Act remedies can only be advertised by special prescription of a doctor. In the town of Zurich the sale of unauthorised remedies even to foreigners is punishable. Although doctors and patients settle their financial relations independently, the Health Authority (1912) (Sanitätsrat) has prepared a scale of fees to serve as a guide to courts in the event of a dispute.

In every district a district medical officer and a veterinary surgeon are appointed. The D.M.O. is the legal doctor of the district. He undertakes vaccination so far as this is not done by private doctors. His annual stipend is 200 francs, with special fees for medico-legal work.

Hospital Organisation

Hospitals are chiefly maintained by the Cantonal Governments, and the Zurich arrangements illustrate the best type of arrangements, which were made by a Cantonal Order dated October 1924.

For inhabitants of the canton the lowest charge to patients is 3 francs a day. This applies to all who pay for themselves, and whose annual income does not exceed 3,500 francs, as well as for those supported by the Poor Fund and other benevolent institutions.

For incomes over 3,500 francs the scale increases with income. Thus, for those whose income is 5,001 to 5,500 francs the daily charge is 5 francs, gradually increasing to 9 francs for those earning over 9,000 francs a year. A reduction of 20 per cent. is made for those staying in the hospital longer than fifty days. For persons earning over 10,000 francs an additional charge of 5 centimes is made for every 1,000 francs extra income. The charges can be made exactly, as the official tax registers are applicable for this purpose, if required. For non-residents higher charges are made.

For patients who elect to be treated in a ward with only one to three beds, the charge varies from 8 to 18 francs for residents, 10 to 22 francs for other Swiss subjects, and for others 18 to 30 francs. These charges include medical attendance. Another class of patients is received who pay 10 to 25 francs a day, and pay separately for medical attendance. For children there are modified charges.

The municipality are authorised to make specially favourable terms with sick benefit societies, with employers of labour who have voluntary systems of insurance, and with accident insurance companies. Special terms may also be made for patients whose cases are useful for clinical education.

Polyclinics.—There are polyclinics for each special department of medicine in Zurich, which, while they are under the control of the municipality, are managed in the main by the medical staff and professors of the University. These polyclinics are intended to give expert assistance to the poorer people, and to serve for the training of medical students and younger medical men. The cost is borne by the municipality in conjunction with the Poor Law section of the Cantonal Ministry. At the clinics are treated poorer people, persons treated under special agreements, military patients, and persons sent by the Accident Insurance Institution; also officials of sickness and care institutions, students of the University and technical schools, and any others whose cases have educational interest.

It does not appear that these arrangements excite adverse criticism from private medical practitioners. Their own patients are received in consultation when this is desired.

MIDWIFERY

Perhaps midwives have a more direct influence on infantile hygiene than any other class of women: and it is satisfactory to note therefore that in Switzerland the training of these women, which formerly lasted only six months, must now occupy one or two years, according to the school in which the training is effected. The conditions of their training and practice in the canton of Zurich include the condition that they must attend at stated intervals a "refresher" course for a fortnight. The district medical officer supervises her work. Each commune settles the rate of remuneration of the midwife. This applies to the poor, for whom the commune pays; for others she can charge a higher fee. The midwife is allowed to give advice to the pregnant; but she must call a doctor if abnormal conditions appear. She is especially forbidden to take any action for "restoration of absent catamenia". She is bound to notify every birth in her practice to the civil authority within three days.

Child Welfare Work

The course of infant mortality from 1905 to 1911 showed no evidence of steady decline. It was 123 per 1,000 births in 1911 and 127 in 1906. In more recent years it has never exceeded 100, and was 61 in 1923. It is noteworthy also that the death-rate per 1,000 births for infants under a month old, which was 48 in 1911, was only 38 in 1922 and 33 in 1923.

A number of social dispensaries, including infant consultations, have been formed; but these are insufficient in number, and consultations for expectant mothers are exceptional.

Primes d'allaitement, bonuses for lactation, have already been mentioned. In St. Gall 41 per cent. of the mothers subsidised by the communal insurance *caisses* have obtained this benefit. In Zurich the municipality makes itself responsible for the charges for accouchements in families in which the income is less than 4,000 francs; and in 1925, 12·5 per cent. of those confined in Zurich benefited by this.

School hygiene on its medical side is not well developed in many parts of Switzerland, but in some large towns there are promising developments. In eighteen towns there are school dental clinics. School doctors usually have visiting nurses associated with them. In most communes few arrangements for medical treatment of scholars exist in those cantons in which there is no school medical insurance, apart from reference to private doctors or hospitals.

Control of Tuberculosis

Mention has been made of the fact that only recently has the Federal Government had power to take part in the struggle against tuberculosis. A new federal law was passed in June 1928, which is on very general lines, as a direct referendum to the people would have been necessary had its terms been more specific. This law makes cases of tuberculosis notifiable throughout Switzerland when the state of the patient and the conditions in which he lives imply danger to others. Evidently the judge on these points

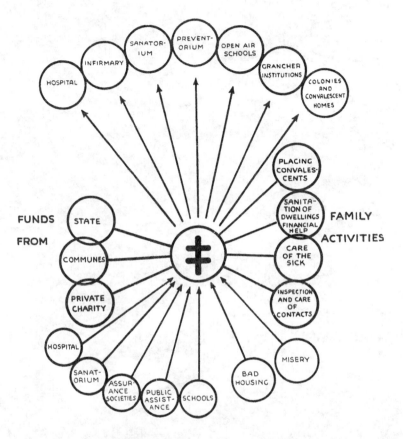

SCHEME OF ACTIVITIES OF THE TUBERCULOSIS DISPENSARY
AT THE POLYCLINIC, LAUSANNE

Facing page 233.

will be the notifying physician: and evidently also such limited notification does not open the way directly for the family and occupational precautions which may be needed, whatever may be the medical decision as to whether the case in question is at the moment one of "open" tuberculosis or not. The Act allots to the cantons which carry out specified anti-tuberculosis work subventions from federal funds of 20 to 25 per cent. for some parts, and 50 per cent. for other parts of this work.

A large amount of anti-tuberculosis work has been undertaken by the cantons, which I can only illustrate by a few examples furnished by Dr. Carrière, the medical head of the Public Health service of the Federation, to whose courtesy I am much indebted. From the documents furnished by him, in supplementation of our conference, much of the information set out in the following pages is derived.

Dr. Carrière's Annual Report for 1927 states that in that year a grant of 1,500,000 francs (25 francs = £1) was given by the Federation in aid of anti-tuberculosis work.

83 leagues and dispensaries received 658,585 francs, or about 24·7 per cent. of their total expenditure;
38 sanatoriums and other establishments for adults received 482,950 francs, or about 8·9 per cent. of their total expenditure;
36 sanatoriums and preventoriums for infants received 158,705 francs, or about 11·5 per cent. of their total expenditure;
73 pavilions and divisions of hospitals for tuberculous patients received 191,417 francs, or 7·3 per cent. of their total expenditure.

The total federal subvention was 1,491,657 francs. This, it will be noted, was before the law of 1928 came into operation.

The giving of these subventions enabled the Federal Government to exercise a measure of control over the administration of cantonal anti-tuberculosis measures.

The scope of activities against tuberculosis is illustrated in the accompanying scheme, showing the plan of work of the tuberculosis dispensary at the polyclinic in Lausanne. The scheme is in part futurist; but it is useful as showing the various directions in which good work is being pursued.

The improvement in habits of the people is illustrated by the fact that federal inspectors of factories have secured a change from cuspidors containing sawdust to cuspidors holding fluid, and that the latter are rapidly becoming unused, owing to the improved habits of the workers.

According to a report by Dr. E. Olivier and others issued by the Swiss Anti-Tuberculosis Association, there are in Switzerland 62 local associations with 127 regional branches. There are 30 tuberculosis dispensaries, which follow the practice of avoiding the domain of the private medical practitioner. Difficulties have arisen in this connection, especially as regards the administration of tuberculin and in pneumothorax cases. As a rule the dispensaries are not conducted by tuberculosis experts, who engage only in the work of the dispensaries. There are a few public health nurses for home visiting from the dispensaries, and the number is increasing.

In 1913 the canton of Vaud adopted legislation empowering a subsidy of 2 francs a day for grave open tuberculosis patients in impoverished circumstances, for whom hospital treatment was not indicated. This power does not appear to have been widely utilised. The extent of hospital treatment for tuberculosis is partially indicated by the fact that for the whole of Switzerland in 1891–95 the percentage proportion of total deaths from tuberculosis which occurred in hospitals was 36·5, in 1906–10 it was 43·3.

CONTROL OF VENEREAL DISEASES

The control of *venereal diseases* varies, as might be anticipated in view of the decentralisation of administration, in each canton, and even in each commune or municipality. There is an active Swiss society for the prevention of venereal diseases, which has done good work. In 1923 it published a valuable study of *Les Maladies Vénériennes en Suisse*, written by Dr. H. Jaeger, of Zurich, which gives the results—much more complete than one could have anticipated—of an inquiry into the number of cases of venereal diseases in the practice of every doctor in Switzerland. The chief value of the return is in giving a minimum idea of the prevalence of venereal disease; in this respect it gives the experience of 75 per cent. of all doctors and 95 per cent. of the specialists in venereal disease, as well as the total experience of polyclinics and anti-venereal dispensaries in the country. During the year of inquiry 4 per 1,000 of the inhabitants of Switzerland, without distinction of age or sex, were treated for venereal disease. The number of persons who contracted venereal disease during the year was 1·73 per 1,000, varying from 5·18 in the canton of Geneva to 0·25 in the canton of Schwyz.

Much educational work by conferences, lectures, and pictures is being carried on. Each medical student receives instruction in venereal disease, but Dr. R. Chable, Professor of the University of Neufchâtel, regards a reform and improvement in medical studies as very necessary in this domain.

In some cantons anti-venereal work is subsidised, as in supporting special clinics and polyclinics at the medical schools of Universities. In Geneva the Red Cross support entirely two special venereal disease dispensaries. In Bâle, Geneva, Lausanne, Zurich, and Neufchâtel there are town dispensaries supported by the commune.

Treatment is given gratuitously to the indigent, but not to all comers, unlike the practice in Great Britain and Belgium.

At Geneva public health nurses visit patients who neglect to continue treatment. At Neufchâtel a letter is sent to the patient in such cases, and sometimes the intervention of the family doctor is solicited. As a rule, however, Dr. Chable states that there is no complaint by the dispensary doctor of premature discontinuance of treatment.

Legislation varies greatly as to conditions of medical practice in the different cantons. There is less trouble with

charlatans than with pharmacists, to whom venereal
patients are very apt to resort when first ill. A serious
obstacle to good work is the fact that some sickness
societies continue to refuse to accord their benefit to
members suffering from venereal disease. This difficulty
was serious also in England, but insurance societies in that
country have now abandoned any such differential rule,
which is contrary to the interest of the community and of
the finances of the insurance society, as well as of the
patient himself.

There appear to be no arrangements for the gratuitous
supply to physicians of special drugs, and no general
system of gratuitous examination of blood or of secretions
for spirochœtes or gonococci; and the struggle against
venereal disease in Switzerland must therefore, in view of
the above short review, be described as in a relatively
early stage of development.

SOCIAL INSURANCES

Cantonal self-government has been associated with many
interesting experiments in social insurance. Only a brief
outline can be given here. For much of my information I
am indebted, by the courtesy of Dr. Carrière, to an unpub-
lished brochure by Dr. A. Lemazure, of Berne. The
information as to school medical insurance has been obtained at personal conferences with Dr. F. Wanner, Chief
of the Health Service of Vaud, and his staff, and from the
many official documents concerning this service which
have been placed at my disposal. I take this opportunity
of thanking Dr. Wanner and the many other officials who
helped in throwing light on their valuable and progressive
work.

Insurance against accidents is compulsory for a number
of industries throughout Switzerland. There were evident
reasons for dealing nationally with industrial accident
insurance; but hesitation was felt in applying compulsion
to this extent for sickness. An early attempt to include
sickness and accident alike on a compulsory insurance

basis, for all persons employed by others, was rejected on referendum by a crushing majority of the people. By the amended legislation of June 1911 power was given to each canton to act according to its own discretion as regards sickness insurance.

Sickness Insurance.—This legislation gives the power to enact compulsory sickness insurance to those cantons wishing this, and authorises federal subsidies for such insurance. In this respect the position is somewhat similar to that in Belgium (up to 1930). The Federal Government subsidises sickness societies (*caisses-maladies*) which fulfil certain legal conditions. The control of these subsidies is in the hands of the Federal Office of Social Assurances, to which this work has been delegated by the Federal Council. The approval thus given by the Federal Government gives these *caisses reconnues* an advantage over less satisfactory organisations. The minimum federal subsidy is 3·50 francs and the maximum 5·50 francs a year for each person insured; but, in addition, there is a subsidy of 20 francs for each accouchement of a member of an approved society, and of 20 francs more to each insured mother who suckles her infant during at least ten weeks. Further federal allowances are made in respect to members who live in mountainous and remote districts; and in such areas subsidies can be given to institutions which aid in diminishing the cost of sickness and accouchements. Free choice of doctors is allowed to the insured person, among those doctors living in his vicinity, but this is subject sometimes to the condition that the societies may arrange terms of attendance on patients with all doctors who are willing thus to agree, and then the insured must accept one of these doctors. The free choice of doctor ceases when the patient goes into a hospital. Cantonal Governments have fixed tariffs for gratuitous attendance on the indigent, under a system of free choice of doctor, and these terms may be accepted by the doctors for the insured. All members of a society must be charged according to the same tariff. The following extracts from the order of August 4, 1922, issued by the

canton of Vaud, give some idea of the payments made by
administrative authorities for medical attendance :—

	Francs.
For each day visit to a patient, including simple dressings or a small operation	3
Same by night	6
For a major operation	20–40
For a visit and certificate of patient's condition ..	5
For an autopsy and report	30
For appearance in a court of justice (half day)	10–20

Doctors must present detailed accounts to the administrative
authority, and if these are not presented at stated times a
reduction of 25 per cent. can be made in the amount payable !
Extra allowances are made for excessive distances.

Midwives are paid 50 francs for an accouchement and
for consecutive care of the mother during ten days.

For twins the fee is increased to 70 francs.

Beyond 2 kilometres an extra allowance of 1 franc per
kilometre is authorised.

It is legally provided that when an insured person is
obliged to leave the locality of the society to which he
belongs he can join another society near his new abode,
and this society cannot refuse to accept him, even though
he be old or actually ill.

Compulsory Sickness Insurance.—In the above instances
sickness insurance has been organised by voluntary societies.
Some cantons have gone further than this. Dr. Lamazure,
in his brochure, states that eight out of the twenty-five
cantons have introduced obligatory sickness insurance
confined to certain groups of the population. In the cantons
of Vaud, Geneva, and Fribourg such compulsory insurance
is restricted to the children in primary schools. In Bâle-ville,
St. Gall, Appenzell, and in Zoug it is restricted to persons
of limited means.

In Berne there is no compulsory sickness insurance, but
in Bâle Dr. Gengou states about 70 per cent. of the entire
population are insured. In the whole of Switzerland at the
end of 1922, approved societies had over a million members,
or more than a fourth of the entire population. Dr. Lamazure

states that in 1922 32 per cent. of the women and 20·5 per cent. of the children in Switzerland were insured. The extent of insurance may be gathered from the federal subsidies, which in 1923 amounted to 5·2 million francs. The total federal subsidies up to that date amounted to 33·8 million francs.

From the point of view of social provision for a chief risk in life the facultative sickness insurance of Switzerland fails for those who most need it—the indifferent and negligent, who are unwilling to pay the periodical charges of insurance. It is this and allied considerations which have led to continued call in Switzerland for universal sickness and other forms of social insurance on a federal basis. This has been made the subject of protracted study by experts at Zurich, and their report recommends insurance for old age and for the dependent survivors of the insured. The progress of such a scheme will be watched with interest.

Scholastic insurance must be made the subject of further remarks, and I take the methods of the canton of Vaud in illustration.

Scholars' Medical Insurance

The law on *l'assurance maladie infantile obligatoire*, as modified in November 1927, may be thus summarised.

This enactment refers first to the original Act introducing this insurance in 1916, which created a cantonal *caisse*, or society, governed by an Administrative Council, containing two councillors of the State (canton), one representative of the medical profession (Dr. Wanner), and one of pharmacy, and a director and secretary. It works autonomously, but is affiliated to the State Council, by which the members of the Administrative Council have been appointed.

The public, mutual, and obligatory character of the *caisse* is set out, and its object—the supply of medical and pharmaceutical care to its members, including hospitalisation when necessary—is defined. The *caisse* functions under the control of the State, and is financially guaranteed by it.

Every child, whatever its age or nationality, who in the canton of Vaud is in attendance at the primary or infant schools, or in private schools assimilated by the Council of State to these, must join the *caisse*. It is the duty of the municipalities of the communes in which the insured reside to see that their names are duly registered.

The *caisse* is entitled under the federal law of 1911 to federal subsidies. The State (canton) shares in the costs of this insurance to an amount equalling the contributions of the Confederation; the State, furthermore, pays the cost of administration of the *caisse*. The State can also pay subventions to those communes which, acting in concert with the *caisse*, organise services of school hygiene.

When in any year the annual expenditure of the *caisse* is greater than its reserve funds, one-third of the deficit is paid by the State.

The *caisse* is divided into communal sections, receiving the local gratuitous administrative help of the communal authorities.

The contributions of the insured must be paid by the parents; in their default this duty falls on the persons who are responsible for supporting the insured. The ultimate responsibility for payment for indigent persons rests with the commune.

In each district school teachers act as local agents for the *caisse*.

The contributions were fixed in 1928 by an order of the Council of the State at 12 francs a year for each child.

> For two children in a family, ten francs each;
> For three children in a family, eight francs each;
> For four children in a family, seven francs each;
> For five children in a family, six francs each.

The benefits received consist of medical care. This care is given by a doctor selected by the parent, and the terms under which this treatment is given may next be summarised as stated in the agreement between the *caisse* and the Medical Society of Vaud, dated March 1922 and modified in December 1927.

The medical attendance is concerned with both sickness and accidents. The *caisse* agrees to entrust the treatment of the insured solely to members of the above society, or to other doctors who adhere to the conditions of the above agreement. The free choice of doctor is accorded within a defined radius. The *caisse* will not pay for treatment carried out by free polyclinics.

When an operation is indicated, this is done at specified hospitals at the expense of the *caisse*. If the parent of the insured wishes to make other arrangements, these are at his expense; but the *caisse* will reimburse him in accordance with a scale set out in the agreement.

The insured must, except in cases of urgency, respect the consultation hours of the doctor.

The doctor is required to exercise every possible economy in his prescriptions. He must make returns, setting out the nature of the malady, etc.; each return must be sent to the *caisse* as soon as his attendance on a given case of illness has ceased.

The *caisse* undertakes to do everything possible to facilitate the medical work, and is desirous, in *entente* with the Medical Society of Vaud, to develop hygienic measures. It also distributes lists of the doctors undertaking the treatment of insured children.

The doctor is only to be called on for home visits which he judges to be necessary. A change of doctors is allowed during the course of an illness in special circumstances.

The chief items of the tariff under the scheme are as follows: they are an advance in most items of 50 per cent. on the tariff adopted in 1914:—

	Francs
Day visit within a radius of 1 kilometre, or as otherwise agreed	3·00
For each kilometre in excess	1·20
Visit of urgency	4·50
Night visit	7·50
Care of several members of a family (each)	1·50
Consultations at doctor's house, ordinary hours	2·00
Consultations at doctor's house, at other hours	3·00
Higher charges for various operations.	

The *caisse* is advised by a medical councillor, who is a member of the Medical Society, but is not appointed by the society. He can be called in by a doctor to consult as to any case among the insured. When required by the *caisse*, the medical councillor examines and reports on any of the insured, especially with regard to hospital treatment. He will do this in consultation with the private doctor. He is especially called on to warn doctors as to excessive visiting, etc.

From the above brief summary it is evident that the organisation of the *caisse* has been carefully developed. The system appears to have worked satisfactorily, except that doctors were dissatisfied with the older scale of payment per attendance. This dissatisfaction reached its climax in May 1926, when the Medical Society denounced the agreement with the *caisse*. Under the agreement the total financial allotment for medical attendance per insured child—out of which fees per attendance were paid—had been 10·50 francs. It was proposed by the *caisse* to increase this to 12 francs, but the doctors refused to accept any agreement making them collectively responsible for loss on their fees per attendance. The struggle reached a stage at which the Council of the State, having been appealed to by the *caisse*, proposed to suspend its work if an agreement could not be reached. A provisional arrangement was then made for a year, and a supplementary budget provided; and the above quoted terms may be regarded as the result of the doctors' demand for higher emoluments.

From October 1926 onwards an epidemic of influenza occurred, and in the following January 62·5 per cent. of the total insured children required medical attendance, which intensified the doctors' objection to limitation of remuneration.

Dr. Wanner's medical report on the working of the *caisse* shows that of 45,529 cases of illness attended by the doctors of the *caisse* in the year 1926–27, 11·3 per cent. were affections of the ears, nose, or throat, about the same proportion were respiratory affections, and more than double this proportion were infectious complaints. Stress is laid on the value of early attendance of the infectious and other sick children under the scheme, and this doubtless is a good point. It is, however, obviously anomalous for the doctor to be attending a school-child in a family to the possible exclusion of other members of the same family who may be suffering similarly. The same objection holds, in large measure, for the English system of adult sickness insurance, in which the wage-earner is the only insured person. In both instances it would be more satisfactory in the interests of health for one doctor to be responsible for the medical care of the entire family.

Other criticisms suggest themselves. The general practitioner is not usually an expert in the treatment of such conditions as errors of eye refraction, adenoids, chronic otorrhœa, ringworm, which for poorer children would be more satisfactorily treated at a school clinic. Some of these conditions may be treated at the expense of the *caisse* by specialists. The *caisse* gives no dental treatment. A few municipalities provide dental treatment independently of insurance. Small charges are made—for instance, 1 franc for a filling, and 50 centimes for an extraction, the money being collected from the parents by municipal officers. By these means about one-fifth of the total cost is recovered.

Payment of doctors under contract by number of medical attendances has not been found altogether satisfactory in other countries. My own judgment would be that a more limited or a more extended system of medical insurance is desirable. On the first plan, a system of school medical insurance would, I think, be preferable which left family practice untouched, but which provided for the skilled treatment of ophthalmic and dental defects, of diseases of the throat, nose, and ear, of tuberculosis, of certain skin diseases, such as ringworm, and of orthopædics, etc., in all of which some form of specialised treatment may be needed. Notwithstanding these fairly obvious criticisms, this method of insuring medical treatment for school children deserves attention and further study. The essential objection to it, I think, is its segregation from adequate medical arrangements for infancy and for the pre-school period of life.

General Review

Switzerland, in view of the preceding review, may well be described as the home *par excellence* of local "Home Rule". Local self-government is probably more thorough in Switzerland than in any other country. In England local authorities carry out duties which directly or indirectly are sanctioned by national legislation; in Switzerland, as in the United States, there is no federal control of the activities of States (cantons), except what is embodied in the formal constitution of the Federation (Federal Government). Within the limits of the canton, the commune, and the municipality, the details of government in Switzerland are much more bureaucratic than in England. In the latter, however skilful and learned they may be, officials are directly and continuously controlled by the representatives of the people.

Two special instances of centralised control in Switzerland may be mentioned in conclusion. The sale of salt has been since 1803 a Government monopoly, and in each canton the conditions of sale and price of this commodity can be controlled by the Grand Council. This monopoly in the first instance was probably a device to secure an easily collected indirect tax. In the light of recent research as to the relation between deficient iodine in the dietary and the occurrence of goitre and cretinism, the monopoly has acquired great public health value; and for the two chief sources from which Swiss salt is derived it has been arranged that all the rough salt supplied for the cuisine shall be iodised, while table salt is left unmedicated. It is not clear that this provision extends to all cantons, but it holds good in some. The subject is being watched carefully by the Swiss Commission on Goitre: and it appears probable that in a few years a very remarkable decline in endemic disease due to thyroid deficiency will be experienced.

The sale of alcohol can be controlled by the Federal Government, which is desirous to act, but great difficulties have been experienced in taking practical steps. There is taxation on spirits, but a stage has been reached at which taxation tends to increase private distillation and the taxation becomes unproductive, and does not control the consumption of spirits. Private distillation is no new thing in Switzerland. Small farmers, and even peasants, distill their "waste sugar" from grapes, and the private manufacture of spirits from fermented cherries is carried on to an enormous extent.

There is much alcoholism in Switzerland. Very active temperance societies exist, and the Federal Government is at present searching for further means of control: but the problem evidently is one of great difficulty, and the great body of peasants will need to be convinced of the evil before legislative reform can hold out hope of practical success.

An initiative in favour of local option for the communes as regards the sale of spiritous liquors only was put to popular vote in May 1929, but was rejected by heavy majorities in nearly all constituencies.

INDEX TO VOLUME I

[See also Table of Contents, page 15]